Keto air fryer cookbook for beginners:

The ultimate recipes guide for cooking amazing dishes with your air fryer. Enjoy a wide variety of foods with suggestions for every meal of the day

JENSON NEWMAN

TABLE OF CONTENTS

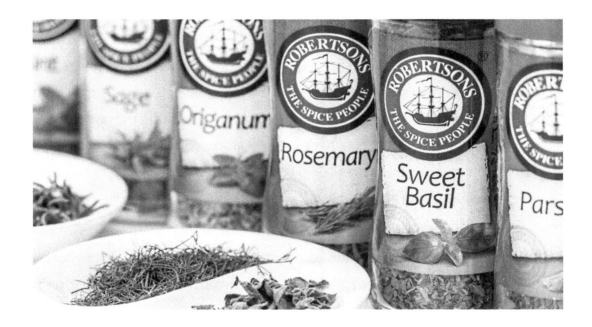

Introduction

U uses up fat bodies called ketones as its main source of energy instead of nder the ketogenic diet, the body is pushed to the state of ketosis wherein it glucose. Unlike other short-lived fad diets, the ketogenic diet has been around for more than ninety years as it was first used to treat patients who suffered from epilepsy. Today, it is still used to minimize the effects of epileptic seizures, but it is also used for weight loss.

People who follow the ketogenic diet limit the intake of carbohydrates to around 20 to 30 net grams daily or 5% of the daily diet. Net grams refer to the number of carbohydrates that remain after subtracting the grams of dietary fiber. Since the carbohydrate intake is limited, dieters are encouraged to consume more fat and protein in amounts of 80% and 20%; respectively.

The ketogenic diet is often referred to as a low-carb diet, but it is important to take note that it [ketogenic diet] is entirely different from the other low-carb diets that encourage protein loading. Protein is not as important as fat is in the ketogenic diet. The reason is that the presence of a higher amount of protein pushes the body to the process called gluconeogenesis wherein protein is converted into glucose. If this happens, the body is not pushed to a state of ketosis. This is the reason why it is so crucial to consume more fat under the ketogenic diet than protein.

When we eat, the carbohydrates found in the food that we consume is converted into a simple sugar called glucose. Alongside converting carbs to glucose, the pancreas also manufactures insulin, which is a hormone responsible for pushing glucose into the cells to be used up as energy.

As glucose is used up as the main source of energy, the fats that you also consume from food is not utilized thus they are immediately stored in the liver and adipocytes (specialized fat cells). Moreover, if you consume too many carbohydrates, the glucose

13

that is not used up is converted into glycogen and is stored in the liver and muscles as standby energy source. If not used up, it is processed and converted to fat and stored all over the body, thus you gain weight.

However, the body is working in a brilliant system that allows us to use up and burn off fats from our body. The ability of the body to produce ketones is part of the millions of years of the human evolution. It protected our ancestors during times of starvation in the past. During periods of famines in the past wherein the body cannot consume carbohydrates over long periods of time, the body uses up fats as a source of energy, as it does in ketosis. This process has helped our ancestors survived for millions of years. Amazing, right?

So, when does ketosis happen? People usually enter the state of ketosis after 3 to 4 days consuming little amounts of carbohydrates. But to undergo the state of ketosis, some people think that you must stop eating altogether—but not with the ketogenic diet. The ketogenic diet bypasses starvation by encouraging you to eat more fats and adequate amounts of protein so that you don't have to undergo starvation. So, what food should you eat? This diet regimen encourages people to consume more fats sourced from healthy and whole food ingredients. That way, the body is pushed to a pure state of ketosis without ever feeling hungry.

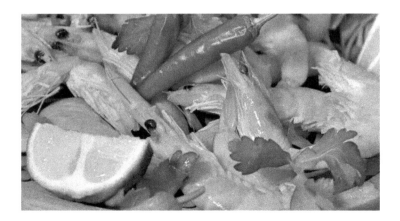

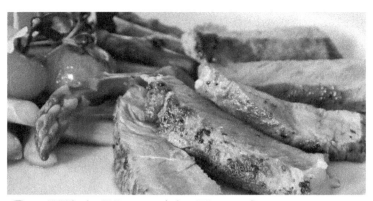

What Can You Do With Your Air Fryer?

I in case you don't, let me introduce you to the wonders of my favorite kitchen f you're reading this cookbook, you probably already know what an air fryer is, but gadget. The air fryer is an "all-in-one" kitchen appliance that promises to replace a deep fryer, convection oven, and microwave; it also lets you sauté your foods. The air fryer is a unique kitchen gadget designed to fry food in a special chamber using superheated air. In fact, the hot air circulates inside the cooking chamber using the convection mechanism, cooking your food evenly from all sides. It uses so-called maillard effect – a chemical reaction that gives fried food that distinctive flavor. Simply put, thanks to the hot air, your foods get that crispy exterior and a moist interior and does not taste like the fat.

Why use an air fryer? I'm asked this question time and time again, so my answer is always the same: it all boils down to versatility, health, and speed. It means that i can "set it and forget it" until it is done. Unlike most cooking methods, there's no need to keep an eye on it. I can pick the ingredients, turn the machine on and walk away – no worries about overcooked or burned food. Another great benefit of using an air fryer is that unlike the heat in your oven or on a stove top, the heat in the cooking chamber is constant and it allows your food to cook evenly. Plus, it is energy-efficient and spacesaving solution.

Is an air fryer worth buying? It is a personal matter. You should keep in mind personal factors such as your kitchen equipment, counter space, budget, cooking preferences, and the size of your family. However, there are numerous benefits you'll get from using an air fryer. Here are the top three benefits of using an air fryer.

Fast cooking and convenience. The air fryer is an electric device, so you just need to press the right buttons and go about your business. It heats up in a few minutes so it can cut down cooking time; further, hot air circulates around your food, cooking it quickly and evenly. Roast chicken is perfectly cooked in 30 minutes, baby back ribs in less than 25 minutes and beef chuck or steak in about 15 minutes. You can use dividers and cook different foods at the same time. The air fryer is a real game changer, it is a cost-saving solution in many ways. I also use my air fryer to keep my food warm. Air fryer features an automatic temperature control, eliminating the need to slave over a hot stove. A digital screen and touch panel allow you to set the cooking time and the temperature according to your recipe and personal preferences.

Healthy eating. Yes, there is such a thing as healthy fried food and the air fryer proves that! The air fryer inspires me every day so that i enjoy cooking healthy and wellbalanced meals for my family. Recent studies have shown that air-fried foods contain up to 80% less fat in comparison to foods that are deep-fried. Deep-fried food contributes to obesity, type 2 diabetes, high cholesterol, increased risk of heart disease, and so on. Plus, fats and oils become harmful under the high heat, which leads to increased inflammation in your body and speeds up aging. Further, these oils release cancer-causing toxic chemicals. Moreover, the spills of fats and oils injure wildlife and produce other undesirable effects on the planet earth.

According to the leading experts, you should not be afraid of healthy fats and oils, especially if you follow the ketogenic diet. Avoid partially hydrogenated and genetically modified oils such as cottonseed oil, soybean oil, corn oil, and rice bran oil. You should also avoid margarine since it is loaded with trans-fats. Good fats and oils include olive oil, coconut oil, avocado oil, sesame oil, nuts and seeds. Air-fried foods are delicious and have the texture of regular fried food, but they do not taste like fat. French fries are only the beginning. Perfect ribs, hearty casseroles, fast snacks, and delectable desserts turn out great in this revolutionary kitchen gadget. When it comes to healthy dieting that does not compromise flavor, the air fryer is a real winner.

The ultimate solution to losing pounds and maintain a healthy weight. One of the greatest benefits of owning an air fryer is the possibility to maintain an ideal weight in an easy and healthy way. The best part is – it doesn't mean that you must give up fried fish fillets, saucy steaks, and scrumptious desserts. Choosing a healthy-cooking technique is the key to success. Air frying requires less fat compared to many other cooking methods, making your weight loss diet more achievable.

Basic keto diet rules

WSo, i decided to change my diet and find an adequate nutrition plan. I knew hat separates a fit person from the couch potato is action. Doing the work!
 – i should find a meal plan that i will follow! Then, i discovered the ketogenic diet and i thought it could be worth considering. Fortunately, i was right! The ketogenic diet is a low-carb, adequate-protein, and high-fat and diet plan. This eating plan involves a significant reduction in carbohydrate intake and replacing it with lean protein and good fats. It means no more junk food, sugar, cereals, and grains. How does it work? On the ketogenic diet, your body produces less glucose and more ketones. Cutting out carbs can lower insulin levels in the blood. Then, your body and your brain accordingly use ketones as energy after you have been on the ketogenic diet for 7 to 8 days. Consequently, you can lose body fat and improve your physical health, cognitive function, and mental performance.

Basically, you should eat protein-rich foods such as fish, seafood, poultry, full-fat dairy products, eggs, and vegetarian keto foods (e.g. Nutritional yeast, tofu, tempeh, shirataki noodles, and seaweed). You should also consume whole foods such as nuts, seeds, and low-carb vegetables. When it comes to the keto beverages, you can consume coffee, tea, sparkling water, and zero carb energy drinks. Foods to avoid on the ketogenic diet include grains, rice, common types of flour, legumes, starchy vegetables, fruits, and sugars. Finally, i can lose pounds and reduce appetite by eating big portions of fatty and high-protein foods. Plus, i am finally free of counting calories and i couldn't be happier than this! When it comes to the keto diet macros, keto requires getting 5% carbs, 20% protein, and 75% fats of total daily calories. Most ketoers stick to this formula as well.

Why i choose the keto diet?

Tsignificant weight loss and improve   d cognitive functions to therapeutic here are numerous science-based benefits of the keto diet. They range from applications.

The ketogenic diet has been shown to reduce bad cholesterol and improve heart health. It can boost brain function and prevent alzheimer's disease, dementia and other brain malfunctions. The ketogenic diet may help treat metabolic syndrome and hypertension. Further, this dietary regimen, with lower insulin levels, may help treat diabetes too. Moreover, studies found that it may slow down the growth of cancer cells. Some clinical trials have proven that you can experience increased memory and mental clarity on the ketogenic diet. In addition to improved mental performance, the stabilization of insulin levels can lead to increased energy levels, too.

How to lose weight on the ketogenic diet?

Calorie counting. Many nutritionists claim that you do not have to count calories on the ketogenic diet. I think it is good advice when it comes to healthy weight maintenance. Otherwise, if you tend to lose weight, you should track your calorie intake. It sounds daunting but, trust me, counting calories and macros is easier than you think. Still, do not go too low and do not consume fewer than 1000 calories per day because it could be counterproductive!

Ketosis can help you reduce hunger. The appetite suppression is one of the greatest advantages of the keto diet. According to experts, ketosis may significantly boost your metabolism. You can practice intermittent fasting to get the most out of keto.

Recent studies have shown that a combination of intermittent fasting and keto-friendly foods can help you maintain ketosis and achieve better results.

Healthy fats. A related point to consider is a type of fat you should consume on a healthy diet. The whole story about fat is confusing, but i think it would be enough to stay away from margarine, processed vegetable oils, and store-bought spreads. I think that many ketoers eat more fat than they need to satisfy their caloric requirements. Keep in mind that high-fat foods can slow down or stop your efforts, even if you only eat healthy fats and very few carbs. It is obvious that you should eat high-quality fat to burn fat, but you should be careful and eat smart. If you eat high-quality fats such as olive oil, coconut oil, avocado and nuts in small amount, your body won't need too many calories; your body needs a small amount of fat to feel full and satisfied. Do not be obsessed with calories and fatty foods. Once you get used to it, you can add a bit fat while continuing to eat fewer carbs; this strategy helps me maintain my weight long term. Plus, i can use my air fryer to prepare fried foods without too much oil. Win-win!

Stay hydrated. Drink enough water to get the most out of the ketogenic diet. On a lowcarb diet, we are skipping various salty carbohydrates, so it's crucial that you increase your intake of essential electrolytes such as potassium, magnesium, sodium, and calcium.

Physical activity. And finally, doing a regular physical activity can help you lose weight faster and make you feel good about yourself. On the ketogenic diet, you can practice low-intensity cardio workouts such as jogging as well as interval training. Doubtlessly, weight lift is one of the best workouts for people on a low-carb diet. Protein-rich foods are building blocks that can help prevent injuries and muscle loss as well as reduce appetite. Plus, keto-friendly foods can help you gain muscle and improve endurance.

Frequently asked questions

I questions about using the air fryer. Below are the frequently asked questions on t is easy to use the air fryer but if you are a first-time user, you must have a lot of how to use the air fryer.

1 – can i cook different foods in the air fryer aside from fried foods?

The air fryer is not limited to cooking only fried foods. You can use it to cook different types of foods like casseroles and even desserts.

2 – how much food do i need to put inside?

Different air fryers tend to have different capacities. If you are not sure how much you need to put in, look for the "max" mark and use it as a guide to fill the basket only to that part.

3 – can i put in more ingredients while the food is being cooked?

Yes. Just open the air fryer so that you can add the ingredients that you want to put in. There is also no need to change the internal temperature as it can stabilize once you close the air fryer chamber.

4 – can i put aluminum or baking paper at the bottom of the air fryer?

Yes. You can use both to line the base of the air fryer. However, make sure that you poke holes so that the hot air can pass through the material and cook food thoroughly.

5 – do i really need to preheat my air fryer?

Preheating the air fryer can reduce the cooking time so you can save energy. Moreover, food comes out crispier. However, if you forgot to preheat, then that is still okay. You can still cook your food, but the quality is not as great as when you preheat the fryer. To preheat the air fryer, simply turn it to the temperature that is needed for cooking and set the timer for 5 minutes. Once the timer turns off, place your food in the basket and continue cooking.

Vegetable

1) Air fryer asparagus

Preparation time: 5 minutes

Cooking time: 8 minutes

Servings: 2

Ingredients

Nutritional yeast

Olive oil non-stick spray

One bunch of asparagus

Directions

Preparing the ingredients. Wash asparagus and then trim off thick, woody ends.

Spray asparagus with olive oil spray and sprinkle with yeast.

Air frying. In your instant crisp air fryer, lay asparagus in a singular layer. Set the temperature to 360°f and set time to 8 minutes.

Nutrition: calories: 17 Fat: 4g

Protein: 9g

2) Crispy ratatouille

Preparation time: 5 minutes

Cooking time: 33 minutes

Serves 4

Ingredients

Kosher salt, for salting and seasoning

1 small eggplant, peeled and sliced ½ inch thick

1 medium zucchini, sliced ½ inch thick

2 tablespoons olive oil

1 cup chopped onion

3 garlic cloves, minced or pressed

1 small green bell pepper, cut into ½inch chunks (about 1 cup)

1 small red bell pepper, cut into ½-inch chunks (about 1 cup)

1 rib celery, sliced (about 1 cup)

1 (14.5-ounce) can diced tomatoes, undrained

¼ cup water

½ teaspoon dried oregano

¼ teaspoon freshly ground black pepper

2 tablespoons minced fresh basil

¼ cup pitted green or black olives (optional)

Directions

Preparing the ingredients. Place a rack on a baking sheet. With kosher salt, very liberally salt one side of the eggplant and zucchini slices, and place them, salted side down, on the rack. Salt the other side. Let the slices sit for 15 to 20 minutes, or until they start to exude water (you'll see it beading up on the surface of the slices and dripping into the sheet pan). Rinse the slices and blot them dry. Cut the zucchini slices into quarters and the eggplant slices into eighths.

Turn the instant crisp air fryer to "sauté", heat the olive oil until it shimmers and flows like water. Add the onion and garlic, and sprinkle with a pinch or two of kosher salt. Cook for about 3 minutes, stirring until the onions just begin to brown.

Add the eggplant, zucchini, green bell pepper, red bell pepper, celery, and tomatoes with their juice, water, and oregano.

High pressure for 4 minutes. Lock the pressure-cooking lid on the instant crisp air fryer and then cook for 4 minutes. To get 4-minutes cook time, press "pressure" button and use the time adjustment button to adjust the cook time to 4 minutes.

Pressure release. Use the quick-release method.

Finish the dish. Unlock and remove the lid. Close the air fryer lid, select broil, and set the time to 5 minutes. Select start to begin. Cook until top is browned.

Stir in the pepper, basil, and olives (if using). Taste adjust the seasoning as needed and serve.

While this vegetable dish is usually served on its own, it's great tossed with cooked pasta or served over polenta.

Nutrition: calories: 149

Fat: 8g

Sodium 55mg

Carbohydrates: 20g Fiber: 8g

Protein: 4g

3)   Avocado fries

Preparation time: 10 minutes

Cooking time: 7 minutes

Servings: 6

Ingredients

1 avocado

½ tsp. Salt

½ c. Panko breadcrumbs

Bean liquid (aquafaba) from a 15-ounce can of white or garbanzo beans

Directions:

Preparing the ingredients. Peel, pit, and slice up avocado.

Toss salt and breadcrumbs together in a bowl. Place aquafaba into another bowl.

Dredge slices of avocado first in aquafaba and then in panko, making sure you get an even coating.

Air frying. Place coated avocado slices into a single layer in the instant crisp air fryer. Set temperature to 390°f and set time to 5 minutes.

Serve with your favorite keto dipping sauce!

Nutrition: calories: 102

Fat: 8g

Sodium 55mg

Carbohydrates: 20g

Fiber: 8g

Protein: 4g

4) Warm quinoa and potato salad

Preparation time: 5 minutes

Cooking time: 45 minutes

Serves 6

Ingredients

¼ cup white balsamic vinegar

1 tablespoon dijon mustard

1 teaspoon sweet paprika

½ teaspoon ground black pepper

¼ teaspoon celery seeds

¼ teaspoon salt

¼ cup olive oil

1½ pounds tiny white potatoes, halved 1 cup blond (white) quinoa

1 medium shallot, minced

2 medium celery stalks, thinly sliced

1 large dill pickle, diced

Directions

Preparing the ingredients. Whisk the vinegar, mustard, paprika, pepper, celery seeds, and salt in a large serving bowl until smooth; whisk in the olive oil in a thin, steady stream until the dressing is creamy.

Place the potatoes and quinoa in the instant crisp air fryer; add enough cold tap water so that the ingredients are submerged by 3 inches (some of the quinoa may float).

High pressure for 10 minutes. Lock the pressure-cooking lid on the instant crisp air fryer and then cook for 10 minutes. To get 10-minutes cook time, press "pressure" button and use the time adjustment button to adjust the cook time to 10 minutes.

Pressure release. Use the quick-release method to bring the pot's pressure back to normal.

Finish the dish. Unlock and open the pot. Close the air fryer lid. Select broil and set the time to 5 minutes. Select start to begin. Cook until top is browned. Drain the contents of the pot into a colander lined with paper towels or into a fine-mesh sieve in the sink. Do not rinse.

Transfer the potatoes and quinoa to the large bowl with the dressing. Add the shallot, celery, and pickle; toss gently and set aside for a minute or two to warm up the vegetables.

Nutrition: calories: 214

Fat: 8g

Sodium 55mg

Carbohydrates: 20g

Fiber: 8g

Protein: 4g

5) Parmesan breaded Preparing the ingredients. To make the **zucchini chips** zucchini chips:

Preparation time: 15 minutes

Cooking time: 20 minutes

Servings: 5

Ingredients

For the zucchini chips:
2 medium zucchinis

2 eggs

⅓ cup breadcrumbs

breadcrumbs

Salt

Pepper

For the lemon aioli:

½ cup mayonnaise
½ tablespoon olive oil
Juice of ½ lemon

1 teaspoon minced garlic

Salt

Slice the zucchini into thin chips (about ⅛ inch thick) using a knife or mandolin.

In a small bowl, beat the eggs. In another small bowl, combine the breadcrumbs, parmesan cheese, and salt and pepper to taste.

Spray the instant crisp basket with cooking oil.

Dip the zucchini slices one at a time in the eggs and then the bread crumb mixture. You can also sprinkle the ⅓ cup grated parmesan cheese breadcrumbs onto the zucchini slices with a spoon.

Place the zucchini chips in the instant Cooking oil crisp air fryer basket, but do not stack.

Air frying. Lock the air fryer lid. Cook in batches. Spray the chips with cooking oil from a distance (otherwise, the breading may fly off). Cook for 10 minutes.

Remove the cooked zucchini chips from the instant crisp air fryer, then repeat step 5 with the remaining zucchini.

Pepper

Directions

and garlic in a small bowl, adding salt and pepper to taste. Mix well until fully combined.

Cool the zucchini and serve alongside the aioli.

Nutrition: calories: 192

Fat: 8g

Sodium 55mg

Carbohydrates: 20g

Fiber: 8g

Protein: 4g

6) Bell peppercorn wrapped in tortilla

Preparation time: 5 minutes

Cooking time: 15 minutes

Servings: 4

Ingredients

To make the lemon aioli:

While the zucchini is cooking, combine the mayonnaise, olive oil, lemon juice,

1 small red bell pepper, chopped

1 small yellow onion, diced

1 tablespoon water

Cobs grilled corn kernels

Large tortillas

Pieces   commercial vegan   nuggets, chopped

Mixed greens for garnish

Directions

Preparing the ingredients. Preheat the instant crisp air fryer to 400°f.

In a skillet heated over medium heat, water sauté the vegan nuggets together with the onions, bell peppers, and corn kernels. Set aside.

Place filling inside the corn tortillas.

Air frying. Lock the air fryer lid. Fold the tortillas and place inside the instant crisp air fryer and cook for 15 minutes until the tortilla wraps are crispy.

Serve with mix greens on top.

Nutrition: calories: 548

Fat: 8g

Sodium 55mg

Carbohydrates: 20g

Fiber: 8g

Protein: 4g

7) Baked cheesy eggplant with marinara

Preparation time: 5 minutes

Cooking time: 45 minutes

Servings: 3

Ingredients

1 clove garlic, sliced

1 large eggplants

1 tablespoon olive oil

1 tablespoon olive oil

1/2 pinch salt, or as needed

1/4 cup and 2 tablespoons dry breadcrumbs

1/4 cup and 2 tablespoons ricotta cheese

1/4 cup grated parmesan cheese

1/4 cup grated parmesan cheese

1/4 cup water, plus more as needed

1/4 teaspoon red pepper flakes

1-1/2 cups prepared marinara sauce

1-1/2 teaspoons olive oil

2 tablespoons shredded pepper jack cheese

Salt and freshly ground black pepper to taste

Directions

Preparing the ingredients. Cut eggplant crosswise in 5 pieces. Peel and chop two pieces into ½-inch cubes.

Lightly grease baking pan of instant crisp air fryer with 1 tbsp olive oil for 5 minutes, heat oil at 390°f. Add half eggplant strips and cook for 2 minutes per side. Transfer to a plate.

Add 1 ½ tsp olive oil and add garlic. Cook for a minute. Add chopped eggplants. Season with pepper flakes and salt. Cook for 4 minutes. Lower heat to 330°f. And continues cooking eggplants until soft, around 8 minutes more.

Stir in water and marinara sauce. Cook for 7 minutes until heated through. Stirring every now and then. Transfer to a bowl.

In a bowl, whisk well pepper, salt, pepper jack cheese, parmesan cheese, and ricotta. Evenly spread cheeses over eggplant strips and then fold in half.

Lay folded eggplant in baking pan. Pour marinara sauce on top.

In a small bowl whisk well olive oil, and breadcrumbs. Sprinkle all over sauce.

Air frying. Lock the air fryer lid. Cook for 15 minutes at 390°f until tops are lightly browned.

Serve and enjoy.

Nutrition: calories: 405

Fat: 21.4g

Protein: 12.7g

8) Spicy sweet potato fries

Preparation time: 5 minutes

Cooking time: 37 minutes

Servings: 4

Ingredients

2 tbsp. Sweet potato fry seasoning mix

2 tbsp. Olive oil

2 sweet potatoes

Seasoning mix:

2 tbsp. Salt

1 tbsp. Cayenne pepper

1 tbsp. Dried oregano

1 tbsp. Fennel

2 tbsp. Coriander

Directions:

Preparing the ingredients. Slice both ends off sweet potatoes and peel. Slice lengthwise in half and again crosswise to make four pieces from each potato.

Slice each potato piece into 2-3 slices, then slice into fries.

Grind together all of seasoning mix ingredients and mix in the salt.

Ensure the instant crisp air fryer is preheated to 350 degrees.

Toss potato pieces in olive oil, sprinkling with seasoning mix and tossing well to coat thoroughly.

Air frying. Add fries to instant crisp air fryer basket. Lock the air fryer lid. Set temperature to 350°f and set time to 27 minutes. Select start to begin.

Take out the basket and turn fries. Turn off instant crisp air fryer and let cook 1012 minutes till fries are golden.

Nutrition: calories: 89

Fat: 14g Protein: 8gs Sugar:3g

9) Creamy spinach quiche

Preparation time: 10 minutes

Cooking time: 20 minutes

Servings: 4

Ingredients

Premade quiche crust, chilled and rolled flat to a 7-inch round   Eggs

¼ cup of milk

Pinch of salt and pepper

1 clove of garlic, peeled and finely minced

½ cup of cooked spinach, drained and coarsely chopped

¼ cup of shredded mozzarella cheese

¼ cup of shredded cheddar cheese

Directions

Preparing the ingredients. Preheat the instant crisp air fryer to 360 degrees.

Press the premade crust into a 7-inch pie tin, or any appropriately sized glass or ceramic heat-safe dish. Press and trim at the edges if necessary. With a fork, pierce several holes in the dough to allow air   circulation   and

        prevent cracking of the crust while cooking.

In a mixing bowl, beat the eggs until fluffy and until the yolks and white are evenly combined.

Add milk, garlic, spinach, salt and pepper, and half the cheddar and mozzarella cheese to the eggs. Set the rest of the cheese aside for now and stir the mixture until completely blended. Make sure the spinach is not clumped together, but rather spread among the other ingredients.

Pour the mixture into the pie crust, slowly and carefully to avoid splashing. The mixture should almost fill the crust, but not completely – leaving a ¼ inch of crust at the edges.

Air frying. Lock the air fryer lid. Set the air-fryer timer for 15 minutes. After15 minutes, the instant crisp air fryer will shut off, and the quiche will already be firm and the crust beginning to brown. Sprinkle the rest of the cheddar and mozzarella cheese on top of the quiche filling. Reset the instant crisp air fryer at 360 degrees for 5 minutes. After 5 minutes, when the instant crisp air fryer shuts off, the cheese will have formed an exquisite crust on top and the quiche will be golden brown and perfect. Remove from the instant crisp air fryer using oven mitts or tongs and set on a heat-safe surface to cool for a few minutes before cutting.

Nutrition: calories: 295

Fat: 14g

Protein: 8gs

Sugar:3g

10) Cauliflower rice

Preparation time: 5 minutes

Cooking time: 20 minutes

Servings: 4

Ingredients   Round 1:

Tsp. Turmeric

1 c. Diced carrot

½ c. Diced onion

2 tbsp. Low-sodium soy sauce

½ block of extra firm tofu

Round 2:

½ c. Frozen peas

2 minced garlic cloves

½ c. Chopped broccoli

1 tbsp. Minced ginger

1 tbsp. Rice vinegar

1 ½ tsp. Toasted sesame oil

2 tbsp. Reduced-sodium soy sauce

3 c. Riced cauliflower

Directions:

Preparing the ingredients. Crumble tofu in a large bowl and toss with all the round one ingredient.

Air frying. Lock the air fryer lid. Preheat the instant crisp air fryer to 370 degrees, set temperature to 370°f, and set time to 10 minutes and cook 10 minutes, making sure to shake once.

In another bowl, toss ingredients from round 2 together.

Add round 2 mixture to instant crisp air fryer and cook another 10 minutes, ensuring to shake 5 minutes in.

Enjoy!

Nutrition: calories: 68 Fat: 14g Protein: 8gs Sugar:0g

11) Buttery carrots with pancetta

Preparation time: 5 minutes

Cooking time: 39 minutes

Serves 4 - 6

Ingredients

4 ounces pancetta, diced

1   medium leek, white and pale green parts only, sliced lengthwise, washed, and thinly sliced

¼ cup moderately sweet white wine, such as a dry riesling

1-pound baby carrots

½ teaspoon ground black pepper

2   tablespoons unsalted butter, cut into small bits

Directions

Preparing the ingredients. Put the pancetta in the instant crisp air fryer turned to the "air fry" function and use the time adjustment button to adjust the cook time to 5 minutes. Add the leek; cook, often stirring, until softened. Pour in the wine and scrape up any browned bits at the bottom of the pot as it comes to a simmer.

Add the carrots and pepper; stir well. Scrape and pour the contents of the instant crisp air fryer into a 1-quart, round, high-sided soufflé or baking dish. Dot with the bits of butter. Lay a piece of parchment paper on top of the dish, then a piece of aluminum foil. Seal the foil tightly over the baking dish.

Set the instant crisp air fryer rack inside and pour in 2 cups water. Use aluminum foil to build a sling for the baking dish; lower the baking dish into the cooker.

High pressure for 7 minutes. Lock the pressure-cooking lid on the instant crisp air fryer and then cook for 7 minutes. To get 7-minutes cook time, press "pressure" button and use the time adjustment button to adjust the cook time to 7 minutes.

Pressure release. Use the quick-release method to return the pot's pressure to normal.

Finish the dish. Close the air fryer lid. Select broil and set the time to 5 minutes. Select start to begin. Cook until top is browned.

Unlock and open the pot. Use the foil sling to lift the baking dish out of the cooker. Uncover, stir well, and serve.

Nutrition: calories: 285

Fat: 14g

Protein: 8gs

Sugar:3g

12) Stuffed mushrooms

Preparation time: 7 minutes

Cooking time: 8 minutes

Servings: 12

Ingredients

2 rashers bacon, diced

½ onion, diced

½ bell pepper, diced

1 small carrot, diced

24 medium size mushrooms (separate the caps & stalks)

1 cup shredded cheddar plus extra for the top

½ cup sour cream

Directions:

Preparing the ingredients. Chop the mushrooms stalks finely and fry them up with the bacon, onion, pepper and carrot at 350 ° for 8 minutes.

When the veggies are tender, stir in the sour cream & the cheese. Keep on the heat until the cheese has melted, and everything is mixed nicely.

Now grab the mushroom caps and heap a plop of filling on each one.

Place in the fryer basket and top with a little extra cheese.

Nutrition: calories: 285

Fat: 14g

Protein: 8gs

Sugar:3g

13) Air fried carrots, yellow squash & zucchini

Preparation time: 5 minutes

Cooking time: 35 minutes

Servings: 4

Ingredients

1 tbsp. Chopped tarragon leaves

½ tsp. White pepper

1 tsp. Salt

1-pound yellow squash

1-pound zucchini

Tsp. Olive oil

½ pound carrots

Directions:

Preparing the ingredients. Stem and root the end of squash and zucchini and cut in ¾-inch half-moons. Peel and cut carrots into 1-inch cubes

Combine carrot cubes with 2 teaspoons of olive oil, tossing to combine.

Air frying. Pour into the instant crisp air fryer basket. Lock the air fryer lid. Set temperature to 400°f and set time to 5 minutes.

As carrots cook, drizzle remaining olive oil over squash and zucchini pieces, then season with pepper and salt. Toss well to coat.

Add squash and zucchini when the timer for carrots goes off. Cook 30 minutes, making sure to toss 2-3 times during the cooking process.

Once done, take out veggies and toss with tarragon. Serve up warm!

Nutrition: calories: 122

Fat: 9g

Protein: 6g

Sugar:0g

14) Tasty hasselback potatoes

Preparation time: 10 minutes

Cooking time: 45 minutes

Servings: 4

Ingredients:

4 potatoes, wash and dry
1 tbsp dried thyme

1 tbsp dried rosemary
1 tbsp dried parsley
½ cup butter, melted
Pepper
Salt
Directions:

Place potato in hasselback slicer and slice potato using a sharp knife.

In a small bowl, mix together melted butter, thyme, rosemary, parsley, pepper, and salt.

Rub melted butter mixture over potatoes and arrange potatoes on air fryer oven tray.

Bake potatoes at 350 f for 25 minutes.

Serve and enjoy.

Nutrition: calories 356

Fat 23.4 g
Carbohydrates 34.5 g
Sugar 2.5 g
Protein 4 g
Cholesterol 61 mg

15) Honey sriracha brussels sprouts

Preparation time: 10 minutes

Cooking time: 15 minutes

Servings: 4

Ingredients:

½ lb. Brussels sprouts, cut stems then cut each in half 1 tbsp olive oil
½ tsp salt
For sauce:
1 tbsp sriracha sauce
1 tbsp vinegar
1 tbsp lemon juice
2 tsp sugar
1 tbsp honey
1 tsp garlic, minced

½ tsp olive oil Directions:

Add all sauce ingredients into the small saucepan and heat over low heat for 2-3 minutes or until thickened.

Remove saucepan from heat and set aside.

Add brussels sprouts, oil, and salt in a zip-lock bag and shake well.

Transfer brussels sprouts on air fryer oven tray and air fry at 390 f for 15 minutes. Shake halfway through.

Transfer brussels sprouts to the mixing bowl. Drizzle with prepared sauce and toss until well coated.

Serve and enjoy.

Nutrition: calories 86

Fat 4.3 g
Carbohydrates 11.8 g
Sugar 7.6 g
Protein 2 g
Cholesterol 0 mg

16) Roasted carrots

Preparation time: 10 minutes

Cooking time: 20 minutes

Servings: 6

Ingredients:

2 lbs. Carrots, peeled, slice in half again slice half
2 ½ tbsp dried parsley
1 tsp dried oregano
1 tsp dried thyme
3 tbsp olive oil
Pepper
Salt
Directions:

Add carrots in a mixing bowl. Add remaining ingredients on top of carrots and toss well. Arrange carrots on air fryer oven pan and roast at 400 f for 10 minutes. After 10 minutes turn carrots slices to the other side and roast for 10 minutes more. Serve and enjoy.

Nutrition: calories 124 Fat 7.1 g

Carbohydrates 15.3 g Sugar 7.5 g

Protein 1.3 g Cholesterol 0 mg

17) Roasted parmesan broccoli

Preparation time: 10 minutes

Cooking time: 5 minutes

Servings: 4

Ingredients:

1 lb. Broccoli florets
¼ cup parmesan cheese, grated
1 tbsp garlic, minced
2 tbsp olive oil
Pepper
Salt
Directions:

Add broccoli florets into the mixing bowl.

Add cheese, garlic, oil, pepper, and salt on top of broccoli florets and toss well.

Arrange broccoli florets on air fryer oven pan and bake at 350 f for 4 minutes.

Turn broccoli florets to other side and cook for 2 minutes more.

Serve and enjoy.

Nutrition: calories 252

Fat 16.4 g
Carbohydrates 8.2 g
Sugar 2 g
Protein 15.3 g
Cholesterol 30 mg

18) Simple baked potatoes

Preparation time: 10 minutes

Cooking time: 40 minutes

Servings: 4

Ingredients:

4 potatoes, scrubbed and washed
¾ tsp garlic powder
½ tsp italian seasoning
½ tbsp butter, melted

½ tsp sea salt Directions:

Prick potatoes using a fork.

Rub potatoes with melted butter and sprinkle with garlic powder, italian seasoning, and sea salt.

Arrange potatoes on instant vortex air fryer oven drip pan and bake at 400 f for 40 minutes.

Serve and enjoy.

Nutrition: calories

163

Fat 1.8 g
Carbohydrates 33.9 g
Sugar 2.6 g
Protein 3.7 g
Cholesterol 4 mg

19) Parmesan green bean

Preparation time: 10 minutes

Cooking time: 5 minutes

Servings: 6

Ingredients:

1 lb. Fresh green beans
½ cup flour
2 eggs, lightly beaten
¾ tbsp garlic powder
½ cup parmesan cheese, grated
1 cup breadcrumbs Directions:

In a shallow dish, add flour.

In a second shallow dish add eggs.

In a third shallow dish, mix together breadcrumbs,   garlic   powder, and cheese.

Coat beans with flour then coat with eggs and finally coat with breadcrumbs.

Arrange coated beans on instant vortex air fryer pan and air fry at 390 f for 5 minutes.

Serve and enjoy.

Nutrition:
calories 257

Fat 8.6 g
Carbohydrates 27.2 g
Sugar 2.6 g
Protein 14.9 g
Cholesterol 75 mg

20) Roasted asparagus

Preparation time: 10 minutes

Cooking time: 9 minutes

Servings: 4

Ingredients:

1 lb. Asparagus, cut the ends
1 tsp olive oil
Pepper
Salt
Directions:

Arrange asparagus on instant vortex air fryer oven pan. Drizzle with olive oil and season with pepper and salt.

Place pan in instant vortex air fryer oven and bake asparagus at 370 f for 7-9 minutes. Turn asparagus halfway through.

Serve and enjoy.

Nutrition: calories 33

Fat 1.3 g
Carbohydrates 4.4 g Sugar 2.1 g
Protein 2.5 g Cholesterol 0 mg

21) Healthy air fryer veggies

Preparation time: 10 minutes

Cooking time: 18 minutes

Servings: 4

Ingredients:

1 cup carrots, sliced
1 cup cauliflower, cut into florets
1 cup broccoli florets
1 tbsp olive oil
Pepper
Salt
Directions:

Add all vegetables in a mixing bowl. Drizzle with olive oil and season with pepper and salt. Toss well.

Add vegetables to the rotisserie basket and air fry at 380 f for 18 minutes.

Serve and enjoy.

Nutrition:
calories 55

Fat 3.6 g
Carbohydrates 5.6 g
Sugar 2.3 g Protein 1.4 g
Cholesterol 0 mg

22) Baked sweet potatoes

Preparation time: 10 minutes

Cooking time: 40 minutes

Servings: 4

Ingredients:

4 sweet potatoes, scrubbed and washed
½ tbsp butter, melted
½ tsp sea salt Directions:

Prick sweet potatoes using a fork.

Rub sweet potatoes with melted butter and season with salt.

Arrange sweet potatoes on instant vortex air fryer drip pan and bake at 400 f for 40 minutes.

Serve and enjoy.

Nutrition: calories 125

Fat 1.5 g
Carbohydrates 26.2 g
Sugar 5.4 g
Protein 2.1 g
Cholesterol 4 mg

23)   Broccoli and cauliflower medley

Preparation time: 10 minutes

Cooking time: 10 minutes

Serving: 2

Ingredients:

1/2 lb. Broccoli fresh
1/2 lb. Cauliflower fresh
1 tablespoon olive oil
1/4 teaspoon black pepper
1/4 teaspoon salt
1/4 teaspoon garlic salt
1/3 cup water Directions:

Toss the vegetable with seasonings and olive oil in a bowl.

Pour 1/3 cup water into the instant pot duo base.

Place the air fry basket inside and spread the vegetables in it.

Put on the air fryer lid and seal it.

Hit the "roast button" and select 10 minutes of cooking time, then press "start."

Once the instant pot duo beeps, remove its lid. Serve.

Nutrition: calories

90

Total fat 7g

Saturated fat 1g

Cholesterol 0mg

Sodium 324mg

Total carbohydrate 7.4g

Dietary fiber 3.1g

Total sugars 2.8g

Protein 3.1g

24) Roasted squash mix

Preparation time: 10 minutes

Cooking time: 40 minutes

Serving: 2

Ingredients:

3 potatoes, cubed

1 red onion, quartered

1 butternut squash, cubed

1 sweet potato, peeled and cubed

1 tablespoon fresh thyme, chopped

2 tablespoons fresh rosemary, chopped

2 red bell peppers, seeded and diced

1/4 cup olive oil

2 tablespoons balsamic vinegar Salt and freshly ground black pepper

Directions:

Whisk rosemary with thyme, vinegar, olive oil, black pepper, and salt in a bowl.

Toss in onion, bell peppers, squash, potatoes, and sweet potato.

Add the vegetables to the instant pot duo.

Put on the air fryer lid and seal it.

Hit the "roast button" and select 40 minutes of cooking time, then press "start."

Toss the roasting vegetables every 10 minutes.

Once the instant pot duo beeps, remove its lid.

Serve.

Nutrition: calories

570

Total fat 26.7g

Saturated fat 4g

Cholesterol 0mg

Sodium 58mg

Total carbohydrate 82.8g

Dietary fiber 11.5g

Total sugars 15.4g

Protein 9.2g

25) Zucchini satay

Preparation time: 10 minutes

Cooking time: 10 minutes

Serving: 2

Ingredients:

2 zucchinis, sliced

2 yellow squash, sliced

1 container mushrooms, halved

1/2 cup olive oil 1/2

onion sliced

3/4 teaspoon italian seasoning

1/2 teaspoon garlic salt

1/4 teaspoon seasoned salt

Directions:

Toss zucchini, squash, onion, and mushrooms in a large bowl.

Whisk olive oil, with italian seasoning, salt, and garlic salt in a small bowl.

Pour this olive oil mixture into the vegetables then toss well.

Spread the seasoned veggies in the air fryer basket.

Set the air fryer basket in the instant pot duo.

Put on the air fryer lid and seal it.

Hit the "air fry button" and select 10 minutes of cooking time, then press "start."

Once the instant pot duo beeps, remove its lid.

Serve.

Nutrition: calories

492

Total fat 51.4g

Saturated fat 7.4g

Cholesterol 1mg

Sodium 22mg

Total carbohydrate 11.8g

Dietary fiber 4.2g Total sugars 5.5g

Protein 4.7g

26) Cauliflower cheese pasta

Preparation time: 10 minutes

Cooking time: 27 minutes

Serving: 4

Ingredients:

9 oz. Shell pasta, cooked and drained

3.5 oz. Unsalted butter

2 bay leaves

1 onion, chopped

3 garlic cloves, crushed

1/2 bunch sage, chopped

1 tbsp plain flour

3 3/4 cups cream

7 oz. Smoked cheese, coarsely grated

1 1/4 cups parmesan, grated 1 large cauliflower, blanched, cut into wedges

1/4 teaspoon nutmeg, grated

Directions:

Place a frypan over medium-high heat and add butter.

Melt it and add garlic, onion, and bay leave then sauté for 5 minutes.

Discard the bay leaves, then stir in flour and sage. Stir cook for 2 minutes.

Slowly add cream, cheese, pasta, and parmesan, then add crumbled cauliflower.

Stir in nutmeg and seasoning, then transfer to the instant pot duo.

Put on the air fryer lid and seal it.

Hit the "bake button" and select 20 minutes of cooking time, then press "start."

Once the instant pot duo beeps, remove its lid.

Serve.

Nutrition: calories

427

Total fat 23.8g

Saturated fat 14.4g

Cholesterol 106mg

Sodium 263mg

Total carbohydrate 43.1g

Dietary fiber 2.5g

Total sugars 2.9g

Protein 12.1g

27) Pumpkin baked gnocchi

Preparation time: 10 minutes

Cooking time: 46 minutes

Serving: 6

Ingredients:

26 oz. Potato gnocchi, cooked

1/3 cup olive oil

16 sage leaves

26 oz. Pumpkin, cut into slices

2 egg yolks

2 ½ cup cream

1/2 teaspoon finely grated nutmeg

3/4 cup coarsely grated mozzarella

3.5 oz. Blue cheese, crumbled

Roasted chopped hazelnuts, to serve

Directions:

Mix pumpkin with 1 tablespoon oil in a bowl.

Stir in egg yolks, cream, gnocchi, half of the sage, half of the blue cheese, nutmeg, cream, and mozzarella.

Spread this mixture in the instant pot duo insert.

Top the casserole with remaining cheese.

Put on the air fryer lid and seal it.

Hit the "bake button" and select 45 minutes of cooking time, then press "start."

Once the instant pot duo beeps, remove its lid.

Heat ¼ cup in a frying pan and add sage. Sauté for 1 minute.

Transfer the fried sage to a plate lined with a paper towel.

Add this fried sage, and nuts to the casserole.

Garnish with sage oil.

Serve.

Nutrition: calories 537

Total fat 30.8g Saturated fat 13g

Cholesterol 122mg Sodium 560mg

Total carbohydrate 50.1g

Dietary fiber 0.8g

Total sugars 0.9g

Protein 17.8g

28) Pumpkin lasagna

Preparation time: 10 minutes

Cooking time: 60 minutes

Serving: 6

Ingredients:

28 oz. Pumpkin, cut into slices

1 bunch sage, chopped

1/2 cup ghee, melted

1 leek, thinly sliced

4 garlic cloves, finely grated

3.5 oz. Kale and cavolo nero leaves shredded

270g semi-dried tomatoes, drained, chopped

17 oz. Quark

2 eggs, lightly beaten Directions:

Mix pumpkin slices with sage leaves, 2 teaspoon salt, 2 tablespoon ghee in a bowl.

Toss leek separately with 2 tablespoon ghee, garlic, and ½ teaspoon salt in another bowl.

Mix kale with 1 teaspoon salt, tomato, and cavolo nero in a bowl.

Now beat eggs with quark and sage in a bowl.

Take a baking pan that can fit into the instant pot duo.

Add 1/3 of the leek mixture at the base of the baking pan.

Top this mixture with a layer of pumpkin slices.

Add 1/3 of quark mixture on top then add 1/3 of kale mixture over it.

Top it with pumpkin slices and continue repeating the layer while ending at the pumpkin slice layer on top.

Place the baking pan in the instant pot duo.

Put on the air fryer lid and seal it.

Hit the "bake button" and select 60 minutes of cooking time, then press "start."

Once the instant pot duo beeps, remove its lid.

Serve.

Nutrition: calories 491

Total fat 29.9g

Saturated fat 16.9g

Cholesterol 147mg

Sodium 1462mg

Total carbohydrate 52.1g

Dietary fiber 9.7g

Total sugars 28g

Protein 14.8g

29) Haloumi baked rusti

Preparation time: 10 minutes

Cooking time: 35 minutes

Serving: 4

Ingredients:

Olive oil, to brush

7 oz. Sweet potato, coarsely grated

10 oz. Potatoes, coarsely grated

10 oz. Carrots, coarsely grated

9 oz. Halloumi, coarsely grated

1/2 onion, coarsely grated

2 tbsp thyme leaves

2 eggs

1/3 cup plain flour

1/2 cup sour cream, to serve

Fennel salad

2 celery stalks, thinly sliced

1 fennel, thinly sliced

1/2 cup olives, chopped

Juice of 1 lemon

1 lemon quarter, chopped 1 teaspoon toasted coriander seeds, ground

Directions:

Toss sweet potato, carrot, potato, onion, halloumi, thyme, flour, and eggs in a bowl.

Spread this mixture in the instant pot duo insert.

Put on the air fryer lid and seal it.

Hit the "bake button" and select 35 minutes of cooking time, then press "start."

Once the instant pot duo beeps, remove its lid.

Prepare   the   salad by
              mixing   its ingredients: in a salad bowl.

Serve the sweet potato rosti with the prepared salad.

Nutrition: calories
462

Total fat 21.1g

Saturated fat 12.8g

Cholesterol 124mg

Sodium 1064mg

Total carbohydrate 43.9g

Dietary fiber 5.9g

Total sugars 8.9g

Protein 23g

30) Celeriac potato gratin

Preparation time: 10 minutes

Cooking time: 63 minutes

Serving: 6

Ingredients:

2 cups cream
1 teaspoon caraway seeds, toasted
1 garlic clove, crushed
1 teaspoon fennel seeds, toasted
2 bay leaves
1/4 teaspoon ground cloves
Zest of 1/2 a lemon
2 teaspoon melted butter
1kg potatoes, peeled

1 cup celeriac, peeled and minced
6 slices prosciutto, torn
3/4 cup fresh ricotta ¼ cup
fontina cheese, grated
Directions:

Add cream, garlic, caraway seeds, cloves, bay leaves, fennel, zest, and cloves to a saucepan.

Stir cook this mixture for 3 minutes then remove from the heat.

Thinly slices potato by passing through the mandolin and spread the potatoes in the insert of instant pot duo.

Top the potato with celeriac, prepared white sauce, prosciutto, and ricotta.

Put on the air fryer lid and seal it.

Hit the "bake button" and select 60 minutes of cooking time, then press "start."

Once the instant pot duo beeps, remove its lid.

Serve.

Nutrition:

calories 399 Total fat 20.3g

Saturated fat 10.9g

Cholesterol 99mg

Sodium 1484mg

Total carbohydrate 23.6g

Dietary fiber 3.8g

Total sugars 4.8g

Protein 31.3g

31) Eggplant pine nut roast

Preparation time: 10 minutes

Cooking time: 66 minutes

Serving: 6

Ingredients:

6 japanese eggplants

2/3 cup olive oil

1 onion, finely chopped

4 garlic cloves, crushed

1 1/2 tbsp sundried tomato pesto

1 teaspoon smoked paprika

14 oz. Can cherry tomatoes

1 teaspoon zaatar, plus extra to serve

2/3 cup vegetable stock

1/2 bunch mint, chopped

2 tbsp toasted pine nuts, roughly crushed

1/4 cup greek yogurt

Juice of 1 lemon Directions:

Add eggplants to the air fryer basket and pour 2 tablespoon oil over them.

Set the air fryer basket in the instant pot duo.

Put on the air fryer lid and seal it.

Hit the "bake button" and select 30 minutes of cooking time, then press "start."

Once the instant pot duo beeps, remove its lid.

Meanwhile, prepare the sauce by sautéing onion with remaining oil in a pan.

After 4 minutes, add garlic to sauté for 2 minutes.

Add tomato, stock, zaatar, paprika and tomato pesto.

Cook this sauce for 10 minutes until it thickens.

Pour this sauce over the eggplant and continue baking it for another 20 minutes.

Mix yogurt with lemon juice, mint, and pine nuts.

Serve the baked eggplants with yogurt.

Nutrition: calories 413

Total fat 25g

Saturated fat 3.7g

Cholesterol 0mg

Sodium 85mg

Total carbohydrate 45g

Dietary fiber 22.1g

Total sugars 27.2g

Protein 9.2g

32) Roasted veggie casserole

Preparation time: 10 minutes

Cooking time: 50 minutes

Serving: 6

Ingredients:

½ head cauliflower, cut into chunks

1 sweet potato, peeled and cubed

2 red bell peppers, cubed

1 yellow onion, sliced

3 tablespoons olive oil

1 teaspoon ground cumin

Salt

Freshly ground black pepper

2 ¼ cups red salsa

½ cup chopped fresh cilantro

9 corn tortillas cut in half

1   can (15 oz.) Black beans, drained

2 big handfuls (about 2 oz.) Baby spinach leaves

2   cups monterey jack cheese, shredded Directions:

Toss the vegetables with olive oil, salt, black pepper, and cumin in a large bowl.

Add these vegetables to the air fryer basket and set it inside the instant pot duo.

Put on the air fryer lid and seal it.

Hit the "bake button" and select 30 minutes of cooking time, then press "start."

Once the instant pot duo beeps, remove its lid.

Transfer the veggies to a baking pan and top it with salsa, tortilla, beans, spinach, and cheese.

Place this pan in the instant pot duo.

Put on the air fryer lid and seal it.

Hit the "bake button" and select 20 minutes of cooking time, then press "start." Once the instant pot duo beeps, remove its lid. Serve.

Nutrition: calories 390 Total fat 20.5g

Saturated fat 8.4g Cholesterol 34mg

Sodium 686mg

Total carbohydrate 38.7g

Dietary fiber 7.4g

Total sugars 9.6g

Protein 15.8g

33) Artichoke mix

Preparation time: 5 minutes

Cooking time: 10 minutes

Servings: 4

Ingredients:

2 cups canned artichoke hearts, halved

1 teaspoon garam masala

1 teaspoon chili powder

2 tablespoons olive oil

A pinch of salt and black pepper

2 tablespoons balsamic vinegar

1 tablespoon dill, chopped

Directions:

In a pan that fits your air fryer, mix the artichokes with the garam masala and the other ingredients and toss.

Put the pan in the air fryer and cook at 400 degrees f for 10 minutes.

Divide between plates and serve.

Nutrition: calories 200 Fat 6

Fiber 2 Carbs 3 Protein 6

34) Roasted beet

Preparation time: 5 minutes

Cooking time: 30 minutes

Servings: 4

Ingredients:

1-pound red beets, peeled and cut into wedges

2 tablespoons avocado oil

A pinch of salt and black pepper

1 teaspoon chili powder

1 tablespoon chives, chopped

Juice of 1 lime

Directions:

In your air fryer's basket, combine the beets with the oil and the other ingredients except the chives, toss and cook at 400 degrees f for 30 minutes.

Divide between plates and serve with the chives on top,

Nutrition: calories 200

Fat 6 Fiber 2 Carbs 3 Protein 6

35)　Potatoes and sauce

Preparation time: 4 minutes

Cooking time: 25 minutes

Servings: 4

Ingredients:

1-pound gold potatoes, peeled and cut into wedges

1 teaspoon turmeric powder

1 teaspoon coriander, ground

2 tablespoons olive oil

A pinch of salt and black pepper

1 cup greek yogurt

1 cup dill, chopped   2

garlic cloves, minced

Directions:

In a bowl, mix the potatoes with turmeric, coriander, oil, salt and pepper and toss.

Put the potatoes in the air fryer's basket and cook at 400 degrees f for 25 minutes.

In a bowl, mix the potatoes with the rest of the ingredients, toss, divide into bowls and serve.

Nutrition:

calories 200

Fat 6

Fiber 2

Carbs 3

Protein 6

36) Balsamic tomatoes

Preparation time: 5 minutes

Cooking time: 20 minutes

Servings: 4

Ingredients:

1-pound cherry tomatoes, halved

¼ teaspoon rosemary, dried

1 teaspoon chili powder

½ cup balsamic vinegar

2 tablespoons olive oil

A pinch of salt and black pepper
Directions:

In your air fryer's basket, combine the tomatoes with the other ingredients, toss and cook at 400 degrees f for 20 minutes

Divide between plates and serve.

Nutrition:

calories 173

Fat 6

Fiber 2

Carbs 3

Protein 6

37) Bacon potato mix

Preparation time: 5 minutes

Cooking time: 30 minutes

Servings: 4

Ingredients:

2 pounds sweet potatoes, peeled and cut into wedges

1 cup bacon, cooked and chopped

2 tablespoons olive oil

1 teaspoon sweet paprika

4 garlic cloves, minced

Juice of 1 lime

Directions:

In the air fryer's pan, mix the sweet potatoes with the bacon and the other ingredients, toss, cook in the air fryer at 390 degrees f for 30 minutes, divide between plates, and serve.

Nutrition:

calories 172

Fat 6

Fiber 2

Carbs 3

Protein 6

38)   Mustard artichokes

Preparation time: 5 minutes

Cooking time: 20 minutes

Servings: 4

Ingredients:

2 cups canned artichoke hearts, drained and halved

2 tablespoons butter, melted

2 tablespoons mustard

3 garlic cloves, minced

½ cup heavy cream

Directions:

In the air fryer's pan, mix the artichokes with the melted butter and the other ingredients, toss, and cook at 400 degrees f for 20 minutes.

Divide between plates and serve.

Nutrition: calories
162 Fat 5

Fiber 3 Carbs 2 Protein 6

39) Lemon beets

Preparation time: 5 minutes

Cooking time: 20 minutes

Servings: 4

Ingredients:

1-pound red beets, peeled and roughly cubed

Fat 6

Fiber 2 minutes.
Carbs 3

Protein 6

Coconut broccoli

Preparation time: 5 minutes

A pinch of salt and black pepper

1 tablespoon lemon zest, grated

1 teaspoon cayenne pepper

1 teaspoon chili pepper

2 tablespoons avocado oil

Juice of 1 lemon

Directions:

In your air fryer's basket, mix the beets with salt, pepper and the other ingredients, toss and cook at 390 degrees f for 20 minutes.

Divide between plates and serve.

Nutrition: calories
200

ingredients, put the pan in the air fryer and cook at 380 degrees f for 30 minutes.

Divide between plates and serve.

Nutrition:
calories 244

Fat 6

Cooking time: 30 minutes

Servings: 4

Ingredients:

1-pound broccoli florets

1 cup coconut cream

1 teaspoon turmeric powder

1 teaspoon cumin, ground

1 tablespoon mustard

½ cup chicken stock

A pinch of salt and black pepper

1 tablespoon parsley, chopped

Directions:

In the air fryer's pan, mix the broccoli
2 shallots, chopped
with the cream, turmeric and the other

1 tablespoon dill, chopped

¼ cup beef stock

Directions:

Fiber 2

Carbs 3

Protein   6

40) Balsamic cauliflower

Preparation time: 5 minutes

Cooking time: 20 minutes

Servings: 4

Ingredients:

1-pound cauliflower florets

1 tablespoon balsamic vinegar

2 tablespoons butter, melted

A pinch of salt and black pepper

In a pan that fits the air fryer, mix the cauliflower with the melted butter and the other ingredients, toss, put the pan in the air fryer and cook at 380 degrees f for 20 minutes.

Divide between plates and serve.

Nutrition:

calories 172

Fat 6

Fiber 2

Carbs 3

Protein 6

41) Broccoli and beets

Preparation time: 5 minutes

Cooking time: 25 minutes

Servings: 4

Ingredients:

1-pound broccoli florets

½ pound beets, peeled and cubed

2 tablespoons avocado oil

1 teaspoon chili powder

½ cup beef stock

½ teaspoon coriander, ground

Salt and black pepper to the taste

½ cup tomato sauce

Directions:

In a pan that fits the air fryer, mix the broccoli with the beets, oil and the other ingredients, put the pan in the fryer and cook at 380 degrees f for 25 minutes.

Divide between plates and serve.

Nutrition: calories 163 Fat 6 Fiber 2

Carbs 3 Protein 6

42) Chili asparagus

Preparation time: 5 minutes

Cooking time: 15 minutes

Servings: 4

Ingredients:

1-pound asparagus spears, trimmed and halved

2 red chilies, minced

2 tablespoons avocado oil

2 tablespoons chili sauce

½ teaspoon sweet paprika A

pinch of salt and black pepper

Directions:

In a bowl, mix the asparagus with the chilies and the other ingredients and rub,

Put the asparagus in your air fryer's basket and cook at 400 degrees f for 15 minutes. Divide between plates and serve.

Nutrition: calories 200 Fat 6 Fiber 2

Carbs 3 Protein 6

43) Parmesan potatoes

Preparation time: 5 minutes

Cooking time: 25 minutes

Servings: 4

Ingredients:

1-pound red potatoes, peeled and cubed

1 cup heavy cream

1 teaspoon turmeric powder

½ cup parmesan, grated

Juice of 1 lime

Salt and black pepper to the taste

2 tablespoons olive oil

Directions:

In the air fryer's pan, mix the potatoes with the cream and the other ingredients, toss, transfer the pan to the machine and cook at 400 degrees f for 25 minutes.

Divide between plates and serve.

Nutrition: calories 200 Fat 6 Fiber 2

Carbs 3 Protein 6

44) Broccoli and carrots

Preparation time: 5 minutes

Cooking time: 20 minutes

Servings: 4

Ingredients:

1-pound broccoli florets

½ pound baby carrots, peeled

2 scallions, chopped

1 teaspoon sweet paprika

½ cup chicken stock

2 tablespoons tomato paste

3 garlic cloves, minced

A pinch of salt and black pepper

1 tablespoon olive oil

Directions:

In the air fryer's pan, mix the broccoli with the carrots and the other ingredients, toss, put the pan in the machine and cook at 400 degrees f for 20 minutes.

Divide between plates and serve.

Nutrition: calories

165 Fat 6

Fiber 2

Carbs 3

Protein 6

45) Butter carrots

Preparation time: 5 minutes

Cooking time: 25 minutes

Servings: 4

Ingredients:

1-pound baby carrots, peeled

3 tablespoons butter, melted

Zest of 1 lime, grated

1 teaspoon chili powder

A pinch of salt and black pepper

1 teaspoon sweet paprika

Directions:

In the air fryer's pan, mix the carrots with the melted butter and the other ingredients, toss, cook at 390 degrees f for 25 minutes, divide between plates and serve.

Nutrition: calories 130, fat 3, fiber 3, carbs 4, protein 8

46) Bell peppers mix

Preparation time: 5 minutes

Cooking time: 20 minutes

Servings: 4

Ingredients:

1-pound red bell peppers, cut into strips

1 teaspoon sweet paprika

1 red onion, sliced

1 cup tomato passata

A pinch of salt and black pepper

1 tablespoon olive oil

1 tablespoon chives, chopped

2 tablespoons lime juice

Directions:

In a pan that fits the air fryer, mix the peppers with the paprika and the other ingredients, toss, put in your air fryer and cook at 360 degrees f for 20 minutes.

Divide the mix between and serve.

Nutrition:

calories 131 Fat 6

Fiber 2

Carbs 3

Protein 6

47) Balsamic carrots

Preparation time: 2 minutes

Cooking time: 25 minutes

Servings: 4

Ingredients:

2 tablespoons olive oil

1-pound carrots, peeled and roughly sliced

2 tablespoons balsamic vinegar

1 teaspoon garam masala

1 teaspoon rosemary, dried

3 garlic cloves, minced Salt

and black pepper to the taste

Directions:

In the air fryer's basket, combine the carrot slices with the oil and the other ingredients, rub and cook at 380 degrees f for 25 minutes.

Divide between plates and serve.

Nutrition:

calories 122

Fat 6

Fiber 2

Carbs 3

Protein 6

48) Creamy beets

Preparation time: 5 minutes

Cooking time: 25 minutes

Servings: 4

Ingredients:

2 pounds baby beets, peeled and halved

1 cup heavy cream

1 teaspoon turmeric powder

A pinch of salt and black pepper

2 tablespoons olive oil

2 garlic cloves, minced

Juice of 1 lime

½ teaspoon coriander, ground

Directions:

In a pan that fits your air fryer, mix the beet with the cream, turmeric and the other ingredients, toss, introduce the pan in the fryer and cook at 400 degrees f for 25 minutes.

Divide between plates and serve.

Nutrition:

calories 135 Fat 6

Fiber 2

Carbs 3

Protein 6

49) Chard and olives

Preparation time: 5 minutes

Cooking time: 20 minutes

Servings: 4

Ingredients:

2 cups red chard, torn

1 cup kalamata olives, pitted and halved

½ cup tomato sauce

1 teaspoon chili powder

2 tablespoons olive oil Salt and

  black pepper to the taste

Directions:

In a pan that fits the air fryer, combine the chard with the olives and the other ingredients and toss.

Put the pan in your air fryer, cook at 370 degrees f for 20 minutes, divide between plates and serve.

Nutrition:

calories 154

Fat 6

Fiber 2

Carbs 3

Protein 6

50) Coconut   mushrooms mix

Preparation time: 5 minutes

Cooking time: 20 minutes

Servings: 4

Ingredients:

1-pound white mushrooms, halved

1 teaspoon sweet paprika

1 red onion, chopped

1 teaspoon rosemary, dried

Salt and black pepper to the taste

2 tablespoons olive oil

1 cup coconut milk

Directions:

In a pan that fits your air fryer, mix the mushrooms with the paprika and the other ingredients and toss.

Put the pan in the fryer, cook at 380 degrees f for 20 minutes, divide between plates and serve.

Nutrition:

calories 162

Fat 7

Fiber 3

Carbs 6

Protein 5

51) Kale and tomatoes

Preparation time: 5 minutes

Cooking time: 20 minutes

Servings: 4

Ingredients:

2 cups baby kale

1-pound cherry tomatoes, halved

1 cup mild salsa

2 scallions, chopped

1 tablespoon olive oil

A pinch of salt and black pepper

2 tablespoons chives, chopped

Directions:

In a pan that fits the air fryer, combine the kale with the tomatoes and the other ingredients and toss.

Put the pan in the air fryer and cook at 380 degrees f for 20 minutes.

Divide between plates and serve.

Nutrition: calories 150 Fat 7 Fiber 3 Carbs 6 Protein 5

Brussels sprouts and tomatoes

Preparation time: 5 minutes

Cooking time: 20 minutes

Servings: 4

Ingredients:

1-pound brussels sprouts, trimmed

½ pound cherry tomatoes, halved

2 tablespoons tomato paste

1 cup chicken stock

½ teaspoon sweet paprika

1 tablespoon olive oil

Salt and black pepper to the taste

1 tablespoon chives, chopped

Directions:

In a pan that fits the air fryer, mix the sprouts with the tomatoes and the other ingredients and toss.

Put the pan in the air fryer and cook at 380 degrees f for 20 minutes.

Divide between plates and serve.

Nutrition: calories

162 Fat 7

Fiber 3

Carbs 6

Protein 5

52) Italian tomatoes

Preparation time: 5 minutes

Cooking time: 20 minutes

Servings: 4

Ingredients:

1-pound cherry tomatoes, halved

1 teaspoon italian seasoning

1 tablespoon basil, chopped

Juice of 1 lime

A pinch of salt and black pepper

4 garlic cloves, minced

2 tablespoons olive oil

Directions:

In a pan that fits the air fryer, mix the tomatoes with the seasoning and the other ingredients, put the pan in the fryer and cook at 380 degrees f for 20 minutes.

Divide between plates and serve.

Nutrition:

calories 173 Fat 7

Fiber 3

Carbs 6

Protein 5

53) Salsa zucchini

Preparation time: 5 minutes

Cooking time: 20 minutes

Servings: 4

Ingredients:

1-pound zucchinis, roughly sliced

1 cup mild salsa

1 red onion, chopped

Salt and black pepper to the taste

2 tablespoons lime juice

2 tablespoons olive oil 1

teaspoon   coriander,

ground

Directions:

In a pan that fits your air fryer, mix the zucchinis with the salsa and the other ingredients, toss, introduce in the fryer and cook at 390 degrees f for 20 minutes.

Divide the mix between plates and serve.

Nutrition:

calories 162 Fat 7

Fiber 3

Carbs 6

Protein 5

54) Green beans and olives

Preparation time: 5 minutes

Cooking time: 20 minutes

Servings: 4

Ingredients:

1-pound green beans, trimmed and halved

1 cup black olives, pitted and halved

1 cup kalamata olives, pitted and halved

1 red onion, sliced

2 tablespoons balsamic vinegar

1 tablespoon olive oil

3 garlic cloves, minced

½ cup tomato sauce

Directions:

In a pan that fits your air fryer, mix the green beans with the olives and the other ingredients, toss, put the pan in the fryer and cook at 350 degrees f for 20 minutes.

Divide the mix between plates and serve.

Nutrition:

calories 162

Fat 7

Fiber 3

Carbs 6

Protein 5

55) Spicy avocado mix

Preparation time: 5 minutes

Cooking time: 15 minutes

Servings: 4

Ingredients:

2 small avocados, pitted, peeled and cut into wedges

1 tablespoon olive oil

Zest of 1 lime, grated

Juice of 1 lime

1 tablespoon avocado oil

A pinch of salt and black pepper

½ teaspoon sweet paprika

Directions:

In a pan that fits the air fryer, mix the avocado with the lime juice and the other ingredients, put the pan in your air fryer and cook at 350 degrees f for 15 minutes.

Divide the mix between plates and serve.

Nutrition:

calories 162 Fat 7

Fiber 3

Carbs 6

Protein 5

56) Spicy black beans

Preparation time: 5 minutes

Cooking time: 20 minutes

Servings: 4

Ingredients:

2 cups canned black beans, drained

1 tablespoon olive oil

1 teaspoon chili powder

2 red chilies, minced

A pinch of salt and black pepper

¼ cup tomato sauce

Directions:

In a pan that fits the air fryer, mix the beans with the oil and the other ingredients, toss, put the pan in the air fryer and cook at 380 degrees f for 20 minutes.

Divide between plates and serve.

Nutrition:

calories 160

Fat 7

Fiber 3

Carbs 6

Protein 5

57) Cajun tomatoes and peppers

Preparation time: 4 minutes

Cooking time: 20 minutes

Servings: 4

Ingredients:

1 tablespoon avocado oil

½ pound mixed bell peppers, sliced

1-pound cherry tomatoes, halved

1 red onion, chopped

A pinch of salt and black pepper

1 teaspoon sweet paprika   ½ tablespoon cajun seasoning

Directions:

In a pan that fits the air fryer, combine the peppers with the tomatoes and the other ingredients, put the pan it in your air fryer and cook at 390 degrees f for 20 minutes.

Divide the mix between plates and serve.

Nutrition:

calories 151

Fat 7

Fiber 3

Carbs 6

Protein 5

58) Olives and sweet potatoes

Preparation time: 5 minutes

Cooking time: 25 minutes

Servings: 4

Ingredients:

1-pound sweet potatoes, peeled and cut into wedges

1 cup kalamata olives, pitted and halved

1 tablespoon olive oil

2 tablespoons balsamic vinegar

A bunch of cilantros, chopped

Salt and black pepper to the taste

1 tablespoon basil, chopped

Directions:

In a pan that fits the air fryer, combine the potatoes with the olives and the other ingredients and toss.

Put the pan in the air fryer and cook at 370 degrees f for 25 minutes.

Divide between plates and serve.

Nutrition:

calories 132 Fat 7

Fiber 3

Carbs 6

Protein 5

Carbs 6 Protein 5

59) Spinach and sprouts

Preparation time: 5 minutes

Cooking time: 20 minutes

Servings: 4

Ingredients:

1-pound brussels sprouts, trimmed and halved

½ pound baby spinach

1 tablespoon olive oil

Juice of 1 lime

Salt and black pepper to the taste

1 tablespoon parsley, chopped

Directions:

In the air fryer's pan, mix the sprouts with the spinach and the other ingredients, toss, put the pan in the air fryer and cook at 380 degrees f for 20 minutes.

Transfer to bowls and serve.

Nutrition: calories 153 Fat 7 Fiber 3

60) Chicken popcorn

Preparation time: 10 minutes

Cooking time: 10 minutes

Servings: 6

Ingredients:

4 eggs
1 1/2 lb. Chicken breasts, cut into small chunks
1 tsp paprika
1/2 tsp garlic powder
1 tsp onion powder
2 1/2 cups pork rind, crushed
1/4 cup coconut flour
Pepper Salt

Directions:

In a small bowl, mix together coconut flour, pepper, and salt.

In another bowl, whisk eggs until combined.

Poultry

Take one more bowl and mix together pork panko, paprika, garlic powder, and onion powder.

Add chicken pieces in a large mixing bowl. Sprinkle coconut flour mixture over chicken and toss well.

Dip chicken pieces in the egg mixture and coat with pork panko mixture and place on a plate.

Spray air fryer basket with cooking spray.

Preheat the air fryer to 400 f.

Add half prepared chicken in air fryer basket and cook for 10-12 minutes. Shake basket halfway through.

Cook remaining half using the same method.

Serve and enjoy.

Nutrition:
calories 265

Fat 11 g
Carbohydrates 3 g
Sugar 0.5 g

Protein 35 g

Cholesterol 195 mg

61) Delicious whole chicken

Preparation time: 10 minutes

Cooking time: 50 minutes

Servings: 4

Ingredients:

3 lbs. Whole chicken, remove giblets and pat dry chicken

1 tsp italian seasoning

1/2 tsp garlic powder

1/2 tsp onion powder

1/4 tsp paprika

1/4 tsp pepper

1 1/2 tsp salt

Directions:

In a small bowl, mix together italian seasoning, garlic powder, onion powder, paprika, pepper, and salt.

Rub spice mixture from inside and outside of the chicken.

Place chicken breast side down in air fryer basket.

Roast chicken for 30 minutes at 360 f.

Turn chicken and roast for 20 minutes more or internal temperature of chicken reaches at 165 f.

Serve and enjoy.

Nutrition: calories 356

Fat 25 g

Carbohydrates 1 g

Sugar 1 g

Protein 30 g

Cholesterol 120 mg

62) Quick & easy meatballs

Preparation time: 10 minutes

Cooking time: 10 minutes

Servings: 4

Ingredients:

1 lb. Ground chicken

1 egg, lightly beaten

1/2 cup mozzarella cheese, shredded

1 1/2 tbsp taco seasoning

3 garlic cloves, minced

3 tbsp fresh parsley, chopped

1 small onion, minced

Pepper

Salt

Directions:

Add all ingredients into the large mixing bowl and mix until well combined.

Make small balls from mixture and place in the air fryer basket.

Cook meatballs for 10 minutes at 400 f.

Serve and enjoy.

Nutrition:

calories 253

Fat 10 g

Carbohydrates 2 g

Sugar 0.9 g

Protein 35 g

Cholesterol 144 mg

63) Lemon pepper chicken wings

Preparation time: 10 minutes

Cooking time: 16 minutes

Servings: 4

Ingredients:

1 lb. Chicken wings 1 tsp lemon pepper

1 tbsp olive oil

1 tsp salt

Directions:

Add chicken wings into the large mixing bowl.

Add remaining ingredients over chicken and toss well to coat.

Place chicken wings in the air fryer basket.

Cook chicken wings for 8 minutes at 400 f.

Turn chicken wings to another side and cook for 8 minutes more.

Serve and enjoy.

Nutrition: calories

247

Fat 11 g

Carbohydrates 0.3 g

Sugar 0 g

Protein 32 g

Cholesterol 101 mg

64) Bbq chicken wings

Preparation time: 10 minutes

Cooking time: 20 minutes

Servings: 4

Ingredients:

1 1/2 lbs. Chicken wings
2 tbsp unsweetened bbq sauce

1 tsp paprika
1 tbsp olive oil
1 tsp garlic powder
Pepper
Salt

Directions:

In a large bowl, toss chicken wings with garlic powder, oil, paprika, pepper, and salt.

Preheat the air fryer to 360 f.

Add chicken wings in air fryer basket and cook for 12 minutes.

Turn chicken wings to another side and cook for 5 minutes more.

Remove chicken wings from air fryer and toss with bbq sauce.

Return chicken wings in air fryer basket and cook for 2 minutes more.

Serve and enjoy.

Nutrition: calories 372 Fat 16.2 g Carbohydrates 4.3 g Sugar 3.7 g

Protein 49.4 g Cholesterol 151 mg

65)   Flavorful fried chicken

Preparation time: 10 minutes

Cooking time: 40 minutes

Servings: 10

Ingredients:

5 lbs. Chicken, about 10 pieces

1 tbsp coconut oil

2 1/2 tsp white pepper

1 tsp ground ginger

1 1/2 tsp garlic salt

1 tbsp paprika

1 tsp dried mustard

1 tsp pepper

1 tsp celery salt

1/3 tsp oregano

1/2 tsp basil

1/2 tsp thyme

2 cups pork rinds, crushed

1 tbsp vinegar

1 cup unsweetened almond milk 1/2 tsp salt

Directions:

Add chicken in a large mixing bowl.

Add milk and vinegar over chicken and place in the refrigerator for 2 hours.

I a shallow dish, mix together pork rinds, white pepper, ginger, garlic salt, paprika, mustard, pepper, celery salt, oregano, basil, thyme, and salt.

Coat air fryer basket with coconut oil.

Coat each chicken piece with pork rind mixture and place on a plate.

Place half coated chicken in the air fryer basket.

Cook chicken at 360 f for 10 minutes then turn chicken to another side and cook for 10 minutes more or until internal temperature reaches at 165 f.

Cook remaining chicken using the same method.

Serve and enjoy.

Nutrition: calories

539

Fat 37 g

Carbohydrates 1 g Sugar 0 g

Protein 45 g Cholesterol 175 mg

66) Yummy chicken nuggets

Preparation time: 10 minutes

Cooking time: 12 minutes

Servings: 4

Ingredients:

1 lb. Chicken breast, skinless, boneless and cut into chunks

6 tbsp sesame seeds, toasted

4 egg whites

1/2 tsp ground ginger

1/4 cup coconut flour

1 tsp sesame oil

Pinch of salt

Directions:

Preheat the air fryer to 400 f.

Toss chicken with oil and salt in a bowl until well coated.

Add coconut flour and ginger in a ziplock bag and shake to mix. Add chicken to the bag and shake well to coat.

In a large bowl, add egg whites. Add chicken in egg whites and toss until well coated.

Add sesame seeds in a large zip-lock bag.

Shake excess egg off from chicken and add chicken in sesame seed bag. Shake bag until chicken well coated with sesame seeds.

Spray air fryer basket with cooking spray.

Place chicken in air fryer basket and cook for 6 minutes.

Turn chicken to another side and cook for 6 minutes more.

Serve and enjoy.

Nutrition:

calories 265

Fat 11.5 g

Carbohydrates 8.6 g

Sugar 0.3 g

Protein 31.1 g

Cholesterol 73 mg

67) Italian seasoned chicken tenders

Preparation time: 10 minutes

Cooking time: 10 minutes

Servings: 2

Ingredients:

2 eggs, lightly beaten

1 1/2 lbs. Chicken tenders

1/2 tsp onion powder

1/2 tsp garlic powder

1 tsp paprika

1 tsp italian seasoning

2 tbsp ground flax seed

1 cup almond flour

1/2 tsp pepper

1 tsp sea salt

Directions:

Preheat the air fryer to 400 f.

Season chicken with pepper and salt.

In a medium bowl, whisk eggs to combine.

In a shallow dish, mix together almond flour, all seasonings, and flaxseed.

Dip chicken into the egg then coats with almond flour mixture and place on a plate.

Spray air fryer basket with cooking spray.

Place half chicken tenders in air fryer basket and cook for 10 minutes. Turn halfway through.

Cook remaining chicken tenders using same steps.

Serve and enjoy.

Nutrition: calories

315

Fat 21 g

Carbohydrates 12 g

Sugar 0.6 g

Protein 17 g

Cholesterol 184 mg

68) Classic chicken wings

Preparation time: 10 minutes

Cooking time: 40 minutes

Servings: 4

Ingredients:

2 lbs. Chicken wings For

sauce:

1/4 tsp tabasco

1/4 tsp worcestershire sauce

6 tbsp butter, melted

12 oz hot sauce Directions:

Spray air fryer basket with cooking spray.

Add chicken wings in air fryer basket and cook for 25 minutes at 380 f. Shake basket after every 5 minutes.

After 25 minutes turn temperature to 400 f and cook for 10-15 minutes more.

Meanwhile, in a large bowl, mix together all sauce ingredients.

Add cooked chicken wings in a sauce bowl and toss well to coat.

Serve and enjoy.

Nutrition:
calories 593

Fat 34.4 g

Carbohydrates 1.6 g

Sugar 1.1 g

Protein 66.2 g

Cholesterol 248 mg

69) Simple spice chicken wings

Preparation time: 10 minutes

Cooking time: 30 minutes

Servings: 3

Ingredients:

1 1/2 lbs. Chicken wings
1 tbsp baking powder, gluten-free
1/2 tsp onion powder
1/2 tsp garlic powder
1/2 tsp smoked paprika

1 tbsp olive oil
1/2 tsp pepper
1/4 tsp sea salt Directions:

Add chicken wings and oil in a large mixing bowl and toss well.

Mix together remaining ingredients and sprinkle over chicken wings and toss to coat.

Spray air fryer basket with cooking spray.

Add chicken wings in air fryer basket and cook at 400 f for 15 minutes. Toss well.

Turn chicken wings to another side and cook for 15 minutes more.

Serve and enjoy.

Nutrition: calories 280

Fat 19 g

Carbohydrates 2 g

Sugar 0 g

Protein 22 g

Cholesterol 94 mg

70) Quick & simple chicken breast

Preparation time: 10 minutes

Cooking time: 22 minutes

Servings: 4

Ingredients:

4 chicken breasts, skinless and boneless
1/2 tsp dried oregano
1/2 tsp dried basil
1/2 tsp dried thyme
1/2 tsp garlic powder
2 tbsp olive oil
1/8 tsp pepper
1/2 tsp salt

Directions:

In a small bowl, mix together olive oil, oregano, basil, thyme, garlic powder, pepper, and salt.

Rub herb oil mixture all over chicken breasts.

Spray air fryer basket with cooking spray.

Place chicken in air fryer basket and cook at 360 f for 10 minutes.

Turn chicken to another side and cook for 8-12 minutes more or until the internal temperature of chicken reaches at 165 f.

Serve and enjoy.

Nutrition:

calories 340

Fat 17.9 g

Carbohydrates 0.5 g

Sugar 0.1 g

Protein 42.3 g

Cholesterol 130 mg

71) Easy & crispy chicken wings

Preparation time: 5 minutes

Cooking time: 20 minutes

Servings: 8

Ingredients:

1 1/2 lbs. Chicken wings

2 tbsp olive oil
Pepper
Salt

Directions:

Toss chicken wings with oil and place in the air fryer basket.

Cook chicken wings at 370 f for 15 minutes.

Shake basket and cook at 400 f for 5 minutes more.

Season chicken wings with pepper and salt.

Serve and enjoy.

Nutrition: calories 192

Fat 9.8 g
Carbohydrates 0 g
Sugar 0 g
Protein 24.6 g
Cholesterol 76 mg

72) Herb seasoned turkey breast

Preparation time: 10 minutes

Cooking time: 35 minutes

Servings: 4

Ingredients:

2 lbs. Turkey breast
1 tsp fresh sage, chopped
1 tsp fresh rosemary, chopped
1 tsp fresh thyme, chopped
Pepper
Salt

Directions:

Spray air fryer basket with cooking spray.

In a small bowl, mix together sage, rosemary, and thyme.

Season turkey breast with pepper and salt and rub with herb mixture.

Place turkey breast in air fryer basket and cook at 390 f for 30-35 minutes.

Slice and serve.

Nutrition: calories 238

Fat 3.9 g
Carbohydrates 10 g
Sugar 8 g
Protein 38.8 g
Cholesterol 98 mg

73) Tasty rotisserie chicken

Preparation time: 10 minutes

Cooking time: 20 minutes

Servings: 6

Ingredients:

3 lbs. Chicken, cut into eight pieces
1/4 tsp cayenne

1 tsp paprika
2 tsp onion powder
1 1/2 tsp garlic powder
1 1/2 tsp dried oregano
1/2 tbsp dried thyme
Pepper
Salt

Directions:

Season chicken with pepper and salt.

In a bowl, mix together spices and herbs and rub spice mixture over chicken pieces.

Spray air fryer basket with cooking spray.

Place chicken in air fryer basket and cook at 350 f for 10 minutes.

Turn chicken to another side and cook for 10 minutes more or until the internal temperature of chicken reaches at 165 f.

Serve and enjoy.

Nutrition:
calories 350

Fat 7 g

Carbohydrates 1.8 g

Sugar 0.5 g

Protein 66 g

Cholesterol 175 mg

74) Spicy asian chicken thighs

Preparation time: 10 minutes

Cooking time: 20 minutes

Servings: 4

Ingredients:

4 chicken thighs, skin-on, and bone-in

2 tsp ginger, grated

1 lime juice

2 tbsp chili garlic sauce

1/4 cup olive oil

1/3 cup soy sauce

Directions:

In a large bowl, whisk together ginger, lime juice, chili garlic sauce, oil, and soy sauce.

Add chicken in bowl and coat well with marinade and place in the refrigerator for 30 minutes.

Place marinated chicken in air fryer basket and cook at 400 f for 15-20 minutes or until the internal temperature of chicken reaches at 165 f.

Turn chicken halfway through.

Serve and enjoy.

Nutrition: calories 403

Fat 23.5 g

Carbohydrates 3.2 g

Sugar 0.6 g

Protein 43.7 g

Cholesterol 130 mg

75) Chicken with broccoli

Preparation time: 10 minutes

Cooking time: 20 minutes

Servings: 4

Ingredients:

1 lb. Chicken breast, skinless, boneless, and cut into chunks

2 cups broccoli florets

2 tsp hot sauce

2 tsp vinegar

1 tsp sesame oil

1 tbsp soy sauce

1 tbsp ginger, minced

1/2 tsp garlic powder

1 tbsp olive oil

1/2 onion, sliced

Pepper Salt

Directions:

Add all ingredients into the large mixing bowl and toss well.

Spray air fryer basket with cooking spray.

Transfer chicken and broccoli mixture into the air fryer basket.

Cook at 380 f for 15-20 minutes. Shake halfway through.

Serve and enjoy.

Nutrition: calories

199

Fat 7.7 g

Carbohydrates 5.9 g

Sugar 1.6 g

Protein 25.9 g

Cholesterol 73 mg

76) Zaatar chicken

Preparation time: 10 minutes

Cooking time: 35 minutes

Servings: 4

Ingredients:

4 chicken thighs

2 sprigs thyme

1 onion, cut into chunks

2 1/2 tbsp zaatar

1/2 tsp cinnamon

2 garlic cloves, smashed

1 lemon juice

1 lemon zest

1/4 cup olive oil

1/4 tsp pepper

1 tsp salt

Directions:

Add oil, lemon juice, lemon zest, cinnamon, garlic, pepper, 2 tbsp zaatar, and salt in a large zip-lock bag and shake well.

Add chicken, thyme, and onion to bag and shake well to coat. Place in refrigerator for overnight.

Preheat the air fryer to 380 f.

Add marinated chicken in air fryer basket and cook at 380 f for 15 minutes.

Turn chicken to another side and sprinkle with remaining zaatar spice and cook at 380 f for 15-18 minutes more.

Serve and enjoy.

Nutrition:

Calories 415
Fat 24.1 g
Carbohydrates 5.2 g
Sugar 1.5 g
Protein 43 g
Cholesterol 130 mg

77) Teriyaki chicken

Preparation time: 10 minutes

Cooking time: 20 minutes

Servings: 6

Ingredients:

6 chicken drumsticks

1 cup keto teriyaki sauce
1 tbsp sesame seeds, toasted
2 tbsp green onion, sliced Directions:

Add chicken and teriyaki sauce into the large zip-lock bag. Shake well and place in the refrigerator for 1 hour.

Preheat the air fryer to 360 f.

Add marinated chicken drumsticks into the air fryer basket and cook for 20 minutes. Shake basket twice.

Garnish with green onion and sesame seeds.

Serve and enjoy.

Nutrition:

Calories 165

Fat 7 g

Carbohydrates 7 g

Sugar 6 g

Protein 16 g

Cholesterol 65 mg

78) Crispy & juicy whole chicken

Preparation time: 10 minutes

Cooking time: 60 minutes

Servings: 8

Ingredients:

5 lbs. Chicken, wash and remove giblets

1/2 tsp onion powder

1/2 tsp pepper

Nutrition:

Calories 430

Fat 8.6 g

Carbohydrates 0.5 g

Sugar 0.1 g

Protein 82.3 g

Cholesterol 218 mg through.

1 tsp paprika

1 tsp dried oregano

1 tsp dried basil

1   1/2   tsp   salt

Directions:

Preheat the air fryer to 360 f.

Mix together all spices and rub over chicken.

Place chicken into the air fryer basket. Make sure the chicken breast side down.

Cook chicken for 30 minutes then turn to another side and cook for 30 minutes more.

Slice and serve.

Spray air fryer basket with cooking spray.

Rub turkey breast tenderloin with paprika, pepper, thyme, sage, and salt and place in the air fryer basket.

Cook for 25 minutes. Turn halfway

Slice and serve.

79) Juicy turkey breast tenderloin

Preparation time: 10 minutes

Cooking time: 25 minutes

Servings: 3

Ingredients:

1 turkey breast tenderloin

1/2 tsp sage

1/2 tsp smoked paprika

1/2 tsp pepper

1/2 tsp thyme 1/2

tsp salt

Directions:

Preheat the air fryer to 350 f.

Nutrition:

Calories 61

Fat 1 g

Carbohydrates 1 g

Sugar 1 g

Protein 12 g

Cholesterol 25 mg

80) Flavorful cornish hen

Preparation time: 10 minutes

Cooking time: 25 minutes

Servings: 3

Ingredients:

1 cornish hen, wash and pat dry

1 tbsp olive oil

1 tsp smoked paprika 1/2 tsp garlic powder

Pepper

Salt

Directions:

Coat cornish hen with olive oil and rub with paprika, garlic powder, pepper, and salt.

Place cornish hen in the air fryer basket.

Cook at 390 f for 25 minutes. Turn halfway through.

Slice and serve.

Nutrition:

Calories 301

Fat 5 g

Carbohydrates 2 g

Sugar 0.5 g

Protein 25 g

Cholesterol 150 mg

81) Chicken vegetable fry

Preparation time: 10 minutes

Cooking time: 15 minutes

Servings: 2

Ingredients:

6 oz chicken breast, boneless and cut into cubes

1/4 tsp dried thyme

1/2 tsp garlic powder

1 tsp dried oregano

1/4 onion, sliced

1/2 bell pepper, chopped

1/2 zucchini, chopped   1 tbsp olive oil

82) Flavorful chicken drumsticks

Preparation time: 10 minutes

Cooking time: 30 minutes

Servings: 4

Ingredients:

8 chicken drumsticks

¼ tsp cayenne pepper

1 tbsp onion powder

1 tbsp garlic powder

1 ½ tbsp honey

1 ½ tbsp fresh lemon juice

1 tbsp worcestershire sauce

¼ cup soy sauce, low sodium

1 tbsp sesame oil

2 tbsp olive oil

½ tsp kosher salt   Directions:

Add all ingredients except chicken in a large mixing bowl and mix well.

Add chicken drumsticks to the bowl and mix until well coated.

Place chicken drumsticks on the instant vortex air fryer rack air fry at 400 f for 15 minutes.

Turn chicken drumsticks to another side and cook for 15 minutes more.

Serve and enjoy.

Nutrition:

Calories 296

Fat 15.8 g

Carbohydrates 11.6 g

Sugar 8.7 g

Protein 26.9 g

Cholesterol 81 mg

83) Gluten-free air fried chicken

Preparation time: 10 minutes

Cooking time: 25 minutes

Servings: 6

Ingredients:

6 chicken drumsticks, rinse and pat dry with a paper towel 1 tsp ginger

1 tsp onion powder

1 tsp garlic powder

1 tsp paprika

1 cup buttermilk

¼ cup brown sugar

½ cup breadcrumbs

1 cup all-purpose flour

½ tsp pepper

1 tsp salt

Directions:

Preheat the instant vortex air fryer using bake mode at 390 f.

Add breadcrumbs, spices, and flour into the zip-lock bag and mix well.

In a bowl, mix together chicken and buttermilk and let sit for 2 minutes.

Now put a single piece of chicken into the zip-lock bag and shake it until chicken is evenly   coated   with breadcrumb mixture. Do this same with remaining chicken pieces.

Spray coated chicken with cooking spray.

Place chicken into the bottom tray of instant vortex air fryer and bake for 25 minutes.

Serve and enjoy.

Nutrition:

Calories 234

Fat 3.8 g

Carbohydrates 31.5 g

Sugar 8.7 g

Protein 17.6 g

Cholesterol 42 mg

84) Parmesan garlic chicken wings

Preparation time: 10 minutes

Cooking time: 21 minutes

Servings: 4

Ingredients:

1 lb. Chicken wings

1 tsp parsley

2 tbsp garlic, minced

¾ cup parmesan cheese, grated

1 tbsp butter, melted

¼ tsp pepper

1 tsp salt

Directions:

Arrange chicken wings on instant vortex air fryer tray and air fry at 400 f for 7 minutes.

Turn chicken wings to the other side and air fry for 7 minutes more.

Turn chicken wings again and air fry for another 7 minutes.

In a mixing bowl, mix together cheese, butter, parsley, garlic, pepper, and salt.

Once chicken wings are done then transfer in mixing bowl and toss well with cheese mixture until well coated.

Serve and enjoy.

Nutrition: calories 398

Fat 20.3 g

Carbohydrates 1.5 g

Sugar 0 g

Protein 45.2 g

Cholesterol 139 mg

85) Healthy   chicken popcorn

Preparation time: 10 minutes

Cooking time: 10 minutes

Servings: 4

Ingredients:

1 lb. Chicken breast, skinless, boneless, and cut into 1-inch pieces 1 egg, lightly beaten

½ tbsp tabasco sauce

1 cup buttermilk

1 tsp baking powder

1 cup all-purpose flour

½ tsp pepper

1 tsp salt

Directions:

Season chicken pieces with pepper and salt.

In a medium bowl, mix together allpurpose flour and baking powder.

In another mixing bowl, mix together egg, buttermilk, and tabasco sauce.

Coat chicken with flour mixture then dip chicken into the egg mixture then again coat with flour mixture.

Place coated chicken pieces on instant vortex air fryer tray. Spray coated chicken pieces with cooking spray.

Air fry chicken popcorn at 400 f for minutes. Turn chicken popcorn to another side and air fry for 5 minutes more.

Serve and enjoy.

Nutrition:

Calories 285

Fat 4.8 g

Carbohydrates 27.6 g

Sugar 3.1 g

Protein 30.7 g

Cholesterol 116 mg

86) Delicious rotisserie chicken

Preparation time: 10 minutes

Cooking time: 50 minutes

Servings: 6

Ingredients:

3 lbs. Whole chicken
¾ tsp garlic powder
¼ cup olive oil
2 cups buttermilk
Pepper
Salt
Directions:

Mix together garlic powder, olive oil, buttermilk, pepper, and salt in a large zip-lock bag.

Add whole chicken in bag. Seal bag and marinate the chicken overnight.

Remove marinated chicken from bag and season with pepper and salt.

Place marinated chicken on the rotisserie spit and inset into the instant vortex air fryer oven.

Air fry chicken to 380 f for 50 minutes or until the internal temperature of chicken reaches 165 f.

Serve and enjoy.

Nutrition:

Calories 537
Fat 25.9 g
Carbohydrates 4.2 g
Sugar 4 g
Protein 68.4 g

87) Cuban chicken wings

Preparation time: 10 minutes

Cooking time: 35 minutes

Servings: 4

Ingredients:

12 chicken wings
2 tbsp water
1 tbsp sazon seasoning
1 tbsp adobo seasoning
1 tsp salt
Directions:

Place chicken wings in a large mixing bowl.

Add remaining ingredients over chicken and toss until chicken is well coated.

Add chicken into the rotisserie basket and place basket into the instant vortex air fryer.

Air fry chicken at 375 f for 35 minutes.

Serve and enjoy.

Nutrition:

Calories 476

Fat 32.1 g

Carbohydrates 16.1 g

Sugar 0 g

Protein 29.2 g

Cholesterol 116 mg

88) Red thai turkey drumsticks in coconut milk

Preparation time: 25 minutes

Cooking time: 23 minutes

Servings: 2

Ingredients:

1 tablespoon red curry paste

1/2 teaspoon cayenne pepper

1 ½ tablespoons minced ginger

2 turkey drumsticks

1/4 cup coconut milk

1 teaspoon kosher salt, or more to taste

1/3 teaspoon ground pepper, to more to taste

Directions

First, place turkey drumsticks with all ingredients in your refrigerator; let it marinate overnight.

Cook turkey drumsticks at 380 degrees f for 23 minutes; make sure to flip them over at half-time. Serve with the salad on the side.

Nutrition: calories 298

Fat 20.3 g

Carbohydrates 1.5 g

Sugar 0 g

Protein 45.2 g

Cholesterol 139 mg

89) Fried turkey with lemon and herbs

Preparation time: 45 minutes

Cooking time: 28 minutes

Servings: 6

Ingredients:

1 ½ tablespoons yellow mustard

1 ½ tablespoons herb seasoning blend

1/3 cup tamari sauce

1 ½ tablespoons olive oil

1/2 lemon, juiced

3 turkey drumsticks

1/3 cup pear or apple cider vinegar

2 sprigs rosemary, chopped

Directions

Dump all ingredients into a mixing dish. Let it marinate overnight.

Set your air fryer to cook at 355 degrees f.

Season turkey drumsticks with salt and black pepper and roast them at 355 degrees f for 28 minutes. Cook one drumstick at a time.

Pause the machine after 14 minutes and flip turkey drumstick.

Nutrition: calories 323

Fat 20.3 g
Carbohydrates 1.5 g
Sugar 0 g
Protein 45.2 g
Cholesterol 139 mg

90) Chicken sausage with nestled eggs

Preparation time: 20 minutes

Cooking time: 17 minutes

Servings: 6

Ingredients:

6 eggs

2 bell peppers, seeded and sliced

1 teaspoon dried oregano

1 teaspoon hot paprika

1 teaspoon freshly cracked black pepper

6 chicken sausages

1 teaspoon sea salt

1 1/2 shallots, cut into wedges

1 teaspoon dried basil

Directions

Take four ramekins and divide chicken sausages, shallot, and bell pepper among those ramekins. Cook at 315 degrees f for about 12 minutes.

Now, crack an egg into each ramekin. Sprinkle the eggs with hot paprika, basil, oregano, salt, and cracked black pepper. Cook for 5 more minutes at 405 degrees f.

Nutrition: calories 221

Fat 20.3 g
Carbohydrates 1.5 g
Sugar 0 g
Protein 45.2 g
Cholesterol 139 mg

91) Parmesan chicken nuggets

Preparation time: 10 minutes

Cooking time: 8 minutes

Servings: 4

Ingredients:

1-pound chicken breast, ground

1 teaspoon hot paprika

2 teaspoon sage, ground

1/3 teaspoon powdered ginger

1/2 teaspoon dried thyme

1/3 teaspoon ground black pepper, to taste

1 teaspoon kosher salt

2 tablespoons melted butter

3 eggs, beaten

1/2 cup parmesan cheese, grated

Directions

In a mixing bowl, thoroughly combine ground chicken together with spices and an egg. After that, stir in the melted butter; mix to combine well.

Whisk the remaining eggs in a shallow bowl.

Form the mixture into chicken nugget shapes; now, coat them with the beaten eggs; then, dredge them in the grated parmesan cheese.

Cook in the preheated air fryer at 405 degrees f for 8 minutes.

Nutrition: calories 346

Fat 20.3 g
Carbohydrates 1.5 g
Sugar 0 g
Protein 45.2 g
Cholesterol 139 mg

92) Tangy and buttery chicken

Preparation time: 20 minutes

Cooking time: 13 minutes

Servings: 4

Ingredients:

½ tablespoon worcestershire sauce

1 teaspoon finely grated orange zest

2 tablespoons melted butter

½ teaspoon smoked paprika

4 chicken drumsticks, rinsed and halved

1 teaspoon sea salt flakes

1 tablespoon cider vinegar

1/2 teaspoon mixed peppercorns, freshly cracked

Directions

Firstly, pat the chicken drumsticks dry. Coat them with the melted butter on all sides. Toss the chicken drumsticks with the other ingredients.

Transfer them to the air fryer cooking basket and roast for about 13 minutes at 345 degrees f.

Nutrition: calories 264

Fat 20.3 g
Carbohydrates 1.5 g
Sugar 0 g
Protein 45.2 g
Cholesterol 139 mg

93) Easy turkey kabobs

Preparation time: 15 minutes

Cooking time: 10 minutes

Servings: 8

Ingredients:

1 cup parmesan cheese, grated

1 ½ cups of water

14 ounces ground turkey

2 small eggs, beaten

1 teaspoon ground ginger

2 ½ tablespoons vegetable oil

1 cup chopped fresh parsley

2 tablespoons almond meal

3/4 teaspoon salt

1 heaping teaspoon fresh rosemary, finely chopped

1/2 teaspoon ground allspice

Directions

Mix all the above ingredients in a bowl. Knead the mixture with your hands.

Then, take small portions and gently roll them into balls.

Now, preheat your air fryer to 380 degrees f. Air fry for 8 to 10 minutes in the air fryer basket. Serve on a serving platter with skewers and eat with your favorite dipping sauce.

Nutrition: calories 360

Fat 20.3 g
Carbohydrates 1.5 g
Sugar 0 g
Protein 45.2 g
Cholesterol 139 mg

94) Turkey breasts with greek mustard sauce

Preparation time: 1 hour 13 minutes

Cooking time: 18 minutes

Servings: 4

Ingredients:

1/2 teaspoon cumin powder

2 pounds turkey breasts, quartered

2 cloves garlic, smashed

½ teaspoon hot paprika

2 tablespoons melted butter

1 teaspoon fine sea salt

Freshly cracked mixed peppercorns, to savor Fresh juice of 1 lemon

For the mustard sauce:

1 ½ tablespoons mayonnaise

1 ½ cups greek yogurt

1/2 tablespoon yellow mustard Directions

Grab a medium-sized mixing dish and combine the garlic and melted butter; rub

this mixture evenly over the surface of the turkey.

Add the cumin powder, followed by paprika, salt, peppercorns, and lemon juice. Place in your refrigerator at least 55 minutes.

Set your air fryer to cook at 375 degrees f. Roast the turkey for 18 minutes, turning halfway through; roast in batches.

In the meantime, make the mustard sauce by mixing all ingredients for the sauce. Serve warm roasted turkey with the mustard sauce.

Nutrition: calories 471

Fat 20.3 g
Carbohydrates 1.5 g
Sugar 0 g
Protein 45.2 g
Cholesterol 139 mg

95) Country-style nutty turkey breast

Preparation time: 30 minutes

Cooking time: 25 minutes

Servings: 2

Ingredients:

1 ½ tablespoons coconut amines

1/2 tablespoon xanthan gum

2 bay leaves

1/3 cup dry sherry

1 ½ tablespoons chopped walnuts

1 teaspoon shallot powder

1-pound turkey breasts, sliced

1 teaspoon garlic powder

2 teaspoons olive oil

1/2 teaspoon onion salt

1/2 teaspoon red pepper flakes, crushed

1 teaspoon ground black pepper
Directions

Begin by preheating your air fryer to 395 degrees f. Place all ingredients, minus chopped walnuts, in a mixing bowl and let them marinate at least 1 hour.

After that, cook the marinated turkey breast approximately 23 minutes or until heated through.

Pause the machine, scatter chopped walnuts over the top and air-fry an additional 5 minutes.

Nutrition: calories 365

Fat 20.3 g
Carbohydrates 1.5 g
Sugar 0 g
Protein 45.2 g
Cholesterol 139 mg

96) Eggs and sausage with keto rolls

Preparation time: 40 minutes

Cooking time: 14 minutes

Servings: 6

Ingredients:

1 teaspoon dried dill weed

1 teaspoon mustard seeds

6 turkey sausages

3 bell peppers, seeded and thinly sliced

6 medium-sized eggs

1/2 teaspoon fennel seeds

1 teaspoon sea salt

1/3 teaspoon freshly cracked pink

peppercorns Keto rolls:

1/2 cup ricotta cheese, crumbled

1 cup part skim mozzarella cheese, shredded

1 egg

1/2 cup coconut flour

1/2 cup almond flour

1 teaspoon baking soda

2 tablespoons plain whey protein isolate

Directions

Set your air fryer to cook at 325 degrees f. Cook the sausages and bell peppers in the air fryer cooking basket for 8 minutes.

Crack the eggs into the ramekins; sprinkle them with salt, dill weed, mustard seeds, fennel seeds, and cracked peppercorns. Cook an additional 12 minutes at 395 degrees f.

To make the keto rolls, microwave the cheese for 1 minute 30 seconds, stirring twice. Add the cheese to the bowl of a food processor and blend well. Fold in the egg and mix again.

Add in the flour, baking soda, and plain whey protein isolate; blend again. Scrape the batter onto the center of a lightly greased cling film.

Form the dough into a disk and transfer to your freezer to cool; cut into 6 pieces and transfer to a parchment-lined baking pan (make sure to grease your hands.

Bake in the preheated oven at 400 degrees f for about 14 minutes.

Serve eggs and sausages on keto rolls.

Nutrition: calories 398

Fat 20.3 g

Carbohydrates 1.5 g

Sugar 0 g

Protein 45.2 g

Cholesterol 139 mg

97) Bacon-wrapped turkey with cheese

Preparation time: 20 minutes

Cooking time: 13 minutes

Servings: 12

Ingredients:

1 ½ small-sized turkey breast, chop into 12 pieces

12 thin slices asiago cheese

Paprika, to taste

Fine sea salt and ground black pepper, to savor

12 rashers bacon

Directions

Lay out the bacon rashers; place 1 slice of asiago cheese on each bacon piece.

Top with turkey, season with paprika, salt, and pepper, and roll them up; secure with a cocktail stick.

Air-fry at 365 degrees f for 13 minutes.

Nutrition: calories 534

Fat 20.3 g

Carbohydrates 1.5 g

Sugar 0 g

Protein 45.2 g

Cholesterol 139 mg

98) Italian-style spicy chicken breasts

Preparation time: 20 minutes

Cooking time: 11 minutes

Servings: 4

Ingredients:

2 ounces asiago cheese, cut into sticks

1/3 cup tomato paste

1/2 teaspoon garlic paste

2 chicken breasts, cut in half lengthwise

1/2 cup green onions, chopped

1 tablespoon chili sauce

1/2 cup roasted vegetable stock

1 tablespoon sesame oil

1 teaspoon salt

2 teaspoons unsweetened cocoa

1/2 teaspoon sweet paprika, or more to taste

Directions

Sprinkle chicken breasts with the salt and sweet paprika; drizzle with chili sauce. Now, place a stick of asiago cheese in the middle of each chicken breast.

Then, tie the whole thing using a kitchen string; give a drizzle of sesame oil.

Transfer the stuffed chicken to the cooking basket. Add the other ingredients and toss to coat the chicken.

Afterward, cook for about 11 minutes at 395 degrees f. Serve the chicken on two serving plates, garnish with fresh or pickled salad and serve immediately.

Nutrition: calories 398

Fat 20.3 g
Carbohydrates 1.5 g
Sugar 0 g
Protein 45.2 g
Cholesterol 139 mg

99) Classic chicken nuggets

Preparation time: 20 minutes

Cooking time: 10 minutes

Servings: 4

Ingredients:

1 ½ pounds chicken tenderloins, cut into small pieces

1/2 teaspoon garlic salt

1/2 teaspoon cayenne pepper

1/4 teaspoon black pepper, freshly cracked

4 tablespoons olive oil

2 scoops low-carb unflavored protein powder

4 tablespoons parmesan cheese, freshly grated

Directions

Start by preheating your air fryer to 390 degrees f.

Season each piece of the chicken with garlic salt, cayenne pepper, and black pepper.

In a mixing bowl, thoroughly combine the olive oil with protein powder and parmesan cheese. Dip each piece of chicken in the parmesan mixture.

Cook for 8 minutes, working in batches.

Later, if you want to warm the chicken nuggets, add them to the basket and cook for 1 minute more.

Nutrition: calories 327

Fat 20.3 g
Carbohydrates 1.5 g
Sugar 0 g
Protein 45.2 g
Cholesterol 139 mg

100) Thai chicken with bacon

Preparation time: 50 minutes

Cooking time: 20 minutes

Servings: 2

Ingredients:

4 rashers smoked bacon

2 chicken filets

1/2 teaspoon coarse sea salt

1/4 teaspoon black pepper, preferably freshly ground

1 teaspoon garlic, minced

1 (2-inch piece ginger, peeled and minced

1 teaspoon black mustard seeds

1 teaspoon mild curry powder

1/2 cup coconut milk

1/2 cup parmesan cheese, grated

Directions

Start by preheating your air fryer to 400 degrees f. Add the smoked bacon and cook in the preheated air fryer for 5 to 7 minutes. Reserve.

In a mixing bowl, place the chicken fillets, salt, black pepper, garlic, ginger, mustard seeds, curry powder, and milk. Let it marinate in your refrigerator about 30 minutes.

In another bowl, place the grated parmesan cheese.

Dredge the chicken fillets through the parmesan mixture and transfer them to the cooking basket. Reduce the temperature to 380 degrees f and cook the chicken for 6 minutes.

Turn them over and cook for a further 6 minutes. Repeat the process until you have run out of ingredients.

Serve with reserved bacon. Enjoy!

Nutrition: calories 612
Fat 20.3 g

Carbohydrates 1.5 g Sugar 0 g
Protein 45.2 g Cholesterol 139 mg

101) Thanksgiving   turkey with mustard gravy

Preparation time: 50 minutes

Cooking time: 45 minutes

Servings: 6

Ingredients:

2 teaspoons butter, softened

1 teaspoon dried sage

2 sprigs rosemary, chopped

1 teaspoon salt

1/4 teaspoon freshly ground black pepper, or more to taste   1 whole turkey breast

2 tablespoons turkey broth

2 tablespoons whole-grain mustard

1 tablespoon butter

Directions

Start by preheating your air fryer to 360 degrees f.

To make the rub, combine 2 tablespoons of butter, sage, rosemary, salt, and pepper; mix well to combine and spread it evenly over the surface of the turkey breast.

Roast for 20 minutes in an air fryer cooking basket. Flip the turkey breast over and cook for a further 15 to 16 minutes. Now, flip it back over and roast for 12 minutes more.

While the turkey is roasting, whisk the other ingredients in a saucepan. After that, spread the gravy all over the turkey breast.

Let the turkey rest for a few minutes before carving.

Nutrition: calories 376

Fat 20.3 g
Carbohydrates 1.5 g
Sugar 0 g
Protein 45.2 g
Cholesterol 139 mg

102) Loaded turkey meatloaf with cheese

Preparation time: 50 minutes

Cooking time: 45 minutes

Servings: 6

Ingredients:

2 pounds turkey mince

1/2 cup scallions, finely chopped

2 garlic cloves, finely minced

1 teaspoon dried thyme

1/2 teaspoon dried basil

3/4 cup colby cheese, shredded

1 tablespoon tamari sauce

Salt and black pepper, to your liking

1/4 cup roasted red pepper tomato sauce

3/4 tablespoons olive oil

1 medium-sized egg, well beaten

Directions

In a nonstick skillet, that is preheated over a moderate heat, sauté the turkey mince, scallions, garlic, thyme, and basil until just tender and fragrant.

Then set your air fryer to cook at 360 degrees. Combine sautéed mixture with the cheese and tamari sauce; then form the mixture into a loaf shape.

Mix the remaining items and pour them over the meatloaf. Cook in the air fryer baking pan for 45 to 47 minutes. Eat warm.

Nutrition: calories 324

Fat 20.3 g

Carbohydrates 1.5 g

Sugar 0 g

Protein 45.2 g

Cholesterol 139 mg

103) Country-style turkey thighs with vegetables

Preparation time: 1 hour 15 minutes

Cooking time: 45 minutes

Servings: 4

Ingredients:

1 red onion, cut into wedges

1 carrot, trimmed and sliced

1 celery stalk, trimmed and sliced

1 cup brussel sprouts, trimmed and halved

1 cup roasted vegetable broth

1 tablespoon apple cider vinegar

4 turkey thighs

1/2 teaspoon mixed peppercorns, freshly cracked

1 teaspoon fine sea salt

1 teaspoon cayenne pepper

1 teaspoon onion powder

1/2 teaspoon garlic powder

1/3 teaspoon mustard seeds

Directions

Take a baking dish that easily fits into your device; place the vegetables on the bottom of the baking dish and pour in roasted vegetable broth.

In a large-sized mixing dish, place the remaining ingredients; let them marinate for about 30 minutes. Lay them on the top of the vegetables.

Roast at 330 degrees f for 40 to 45 minutes.

Nutrition: calories 324

Fat 20.3 g

Carbohydrates 1.5 g

Sugar 0 g

Protein 45.2 g

Cholesterol 139 mg

104) Aromatic turkey breast with mustard

Preparation time: 1 hour

Cooking time: 45 minutes

Servings: 4

Ingredients:

1/2 teaspoon dried thyme

1 ½ pounds turkey breasts

1/2 teaspoon dried sage

3 whole star anise

1 ½ tablespoons olive oil

1 ½ tablespoons hot mustard

1 teaspoon smoked cayenne pepper

1 teaspoon fine sea salt

Directions

Set your air fryer to cook at 365 degrees f.

Brush the turkey breast with olive oil and sprinkle with seasonings.

Cook at 365 degrees f for 45 minutes, turning twice. Now, pause the machine and spread the cooked breast with the hot mustard.

Air-fry for 6 to 8 more minutes. Let it rest before slicing and serving.

Nutrition: calories 321

Fat 20.3 g

Carbohydrates 1.5 g

Sugar 0 g

Protein 45.2 g

Cholesterol 139 mg

105) Rustic turkey breasts

Preparation time: 50 minutes marinating time

Cooking time: 48 minutes

Servings: 4

Ingredients:

1 ½ pounds turkey breasts, boneless and skinless

1/2 palmful chopped fresh sage leaves

1 ½ tablespoons freshly squeezed lemon juice

1/3 teaspoon dry mustard

1/3 cup dry white wine

3 cloves garlic, minced

2 leeks, cut into thick slices

1/2 teaspoon smoked paprika

2 tablespoons olive oil

Directions

Combine sage leaves, lemon juice, mustard, garlic, and paprika in a smallsized mixing bowl; mix thoroughly until everything is well combined.

Then, smear this mixture on the turkey breast. Add white wine and let it marinate about 2 hours.

Transfer to the air fryer cooking basket along with the leeks. Drizzle olive oil over everything.

Bake at 375 degrees f for 48 minutes, turning once or twice.

Nutrition: calories 389

Fat 20.3 g
Carbohydrates 1.5 g
Sugar 0 g
Protein 45.2 g
Cholesterol 139 mg

Pork

106) Pork shoulder chops with soy sauce, maple syrup, and carrots

Preparation time: 5 minutes

pressure: 40 minutes   broil: 7

minutes   total: 52 minutes

pressure level: high release:

natural Serves 6

Ingredients

1 tablespoon bacon fat

3 pounds bone-in pork shoulder chops, each ½ to ¾ inch thick 6 medium carrots

3 medium garlic cloves

⅓ cup soy sauce

⅓ cup maple syrup

⅓ cup chicken broth

½ teaspoon ground black pepper

Directions

Preparing the ingredients. Melt the bacon fat in an instant crisp air fryer, turned to the sauté function. Add about half the chops and brown well, turning once, about 5 minutes. Transfer these to a large bowl and brown the remaining chops.

Stir the carrots and garlic into the pot; cook for 1 minute, constantly stirring. Pour in the soy sauce, maple syrup, and broth, stirring to dissolve the maple syrup and to get up any browned bits on the bottom of the pot. Stir in the pepper. Return the shoulder chops and their juices to the pot. Stir to coat them in the sauce.

High pressure for 40 minutes. Lock the pressure-cooking lid on the instant crisp air fryer and then cook for 40 minutes.

To get 40-minutes cook time, press "pressure" button and use the time adjustment button to adjust the cook time to 40 minutes.

Pressure release. Let the pressure to come down naturally for at least 14 to 16 minutes, then quick release any pressure left in the pot.

Finish the dish. Close air fryer lid and select broil, set time to 7 minutes.

Transfer the chops, carrots, and garlic cloves to a large serving bowl. Skim the fat off the sauce and ladle it over the servings.

Nutrition: calories 291

Fat 23 g
Carbohydrates 3 g
Sugar 0 g
Protein 52 g

Cholesterol 165 mg

107) Apricot glazed pork tenderloins

Preparation time: 5 minutes

cooking time: 30 minutes

total: 35 minutes   Servings: 3

Ingredients

1 teaspoon salt

1/2 teaspoon pepper

1-lb pork tenderloin

2 tablespoons minced fresh rosemary or 1 tablespoon dried rosemary, crushed

2 tablespoons olive oil, divided

Garlic cloves, minced

Apricot glaze ingredients

1 cup apricot preserves

Garlic cloves, minced   4 tablespoons lemon juice

Directions:

Preparing the ingredients. Mix well pepper, salt, garlic, oil, and rosemary.

Brush all over pork. If needed cut pork crosswise in half to fit in instant crisp air fryer.

Lightly grease baking pan of instant crisp air fryer with cooking spray. Add pork.

Air frying. Lock the air fryer lid. For 3 minutes per side, brown pork in a preheated 390°f instant crisp air fryer.

Meanwhile, mix well all glaze ingredients in a small bowl. Baste pork every 5 minutes.

Cook for 20 minutes at 330°f.

Serve and enjoy.

Nutrition: calories 291

Fat 23 g

Carbohydrates 3 g

Sugar 0 g

Protein 52 g

Cholesterol 165 mg

108) Barbecue flavored pork ribs

Preparation time: 5 minutes

cooking time: 15 minutes

total: 25 minutes   Servings: 6

Ingredients

¼ cup honey, divided

¾ cup bbq sauce

Tablespoons tomato ketchup

1 tablespoon worcestershire sauce

1 tablespoon soy sauce

½ teaspoon garlic powder

Freshly ground white pepper, to taste

1¾ pound pork ribs

Directions:

Preparing the ingredients. In a large bowl, mix together 3 tablespoons of honey and remaining ingredients except pork ribs.

Refrigerate to marinate for about 20 minutes.

Preheat the instant crisp air fryer to 355 degrees f.

Place the ribs in an instant crisp air fryer basket.

Air frying. Lock the air fryer lid. Cook for about 13 minutes.

Remove the ribs from the instant crisp air fryer and coat with remaining honey.

Serve hot.

Nutrition: calories 311

Fat 23 g
Carbohydrates 3 g
Sugar 0 g
Protein 52 g
Cholesterol 165 mg

109) Rustic pork ribs

Preparation time: 5 minutes

cooking time: 15 minutes

total: 25 minutes   Servings: 4

Ingredients

1 rack of pork ribs

Tablespoons dry red wine   1

tablespoon soy sauce

1/2 teaspoon dried thyme

1/2 teaspoon onion powder

1/2 teaspoon garlic powder

1/2 teaspoon ground black pepper

1 teaspoon smoke salt

1 tablespoon cornstarch

1/2 teaspoon olive oil

Directions:

Preparing the ingredients. Begin by preheating your instant crisp air fryer to 390 degrees f. Place all ingredients in a mixing bowl and let them marinate at least 1 hour.

Air frying. Lock the air fryer lid. Cook the marinated ribs approximately 25 minutes at 390 degrees f.

Serve hot.

Nutrition: calories 213

Fat 23 g
Carbohydrates 3 g
Sugar 0 g
Protein 52 g
Cholesterol 165 mg

110) Fried pork quesadilla

Preparation time: 10 minutes

cooking time: 12 minutes

total: 22 minutes   Servings: 2

Ingredients

Two 6-inch corn or flour tortilla shells

1   medium-sized   pork   shoulder, approximately 4 ounces, sliced

½ medium-sized white onion, sliced

½ medium-sized red pepper, sliced

½ medium sized green pepper, sliced

½ medium sized yellow pepper, sliced

¼ cup of shredded pepper-jack cheese

¼ cup of shredded mozzarella cheese

Directions:

Preparing the ingredients. Preheat the instant crisp air fryer to 350 degrees. Close air fryer lid and select broil, set time to 20 minutes. Grill the pork, onion, and peppers in foil in the same pan, allowing the moisture from the vegetables and the juice from the pork mingle together. After 20 minutes, remove pork and vegetables in foil. While they're cooling, sprinkle half the shredded cheese over one of the tortillas, then cover with the pieces of pork, onions, and peppers, and then layer on the rest of the shredded cheese. Top with the second tortilla. Place directly on hot surface of the instant crisp air fryer basket.

Air frying. Lock the air fryer lid. Set the instant crisp air fryer timer for 6 minutes. After 6 minutes, when the instant crisp air fryer shuts off, flip the tortillas onto the other side with a spatula; the cheese should be melted enough that it won't fall apart, but be careful anyway not to spill any toppings!

Reset the instant crisp air fryer to 350 degrees for another 6 minutes.

After 6 minutes, when the instant crisp air fryer shuts off, the tortillas should be browned and crisp, and the pork, onion, peppers and cheese will be crispy and hot and delicious. Remove with tongs and let sit on a serving plate to cool for a few minutes before slicing.

Nutrition: calories 324

Fat 23 g
Carbohydrates 3 g
Sugar 0 g
Protein 52 g
Cholesterol 165 mg

111) Keto parmesan crusted pork chops

Preparation time: 10 minutes

cooking time: 15 minutes

total: 25 minutes   Servings: 8

Ingredients

Tbsp. Grated parmesan cheese

1 c. Pork rind crumbs

2 beaten eggs

¼ tsp. Chili powder

½ tsp. Onion powder

1 tsp. Smoked paprika

¼ tsp. Pepper

½ tsp. Salt

4-6 thick boneless pork chops

Directions:

Preparing the ingredients. Ensure your instant crisp air fryer is preheated to 400 degrees.

With pepper and salt, season both sides of pork chops.

In a food processor, pulse pork rinds into crumbs. Mix crumbs with other seasonings.

Beat eggs and add to another bowl.

Dip pork chops into eggs then into pork rind crumb mixture.

Air frying. Spray down instant crisp air fryer with olive oil and add pork chops to the basket. Lock the air fryer lid.

Set temperature to 400°f and set time to 15 minutes.

Nutrition: calories 421

Fat 23 g
Carbohydrates 3 g
Sugar 0 g
Protein 52 g
Cholesterol 165 mg

112) Pork wonton wonderful

Preparation time: 10 minutes

cooking time: 25 minutes

total: 35 minutes   Servings: 3

Ingredients

8 wanton wrappers (leas a brand works great, though any will do)

Ounces of raw minced pork

1 medium-sized green apple

1 cup of water, for wetting the wanton wrappers

1 tablespoon of vegetable oil

½ tablespoon of oyster sauce

1 tablespoon of soy sauce Large pinch

of ground white pepper Directions:

Preparing the ingredients. Cover the basket of the instant crisp air fryer with a lining of tin foil, leaving the edges uncovered to allow air to circulate through the basket. Preheat the instant crisp air fryer to 350 degrees.

In a small mixing bowl, combine the oyster sauce, soy sauce, and white pepper, then add in the minced pork and stir thoroughly. Cover and set in the fridge to marinate for at least 15 minutes. Core the apple, and slice into small cubes – smaller than bite-sized chunks.

Add the apples to the marinating meat mixture and combine thoroughly. Spread the wonton wrappers, and fill each with a large spoonful of the filling. Wrap the wontons into triangles, so that the wrappers fully cover the filling, and seal with a drop of the water.

Coat each filled and wrapped wonton thoroughly with the vegetable oil, to help ensure a nice crispy fry. Place the wontons on the foil-lined air-fryer basket.

Air frying. Lock the air fryer lid. Set the instant crisp air fryer timer to 25 minutes. Halfway through cooking time, shake the handle of the instant crisp air fryer basket vigorously to jostle the wontons and ensure even frying. After 25 minutes, when the instant crisp air fryer shuts off, the wontons will be crispy golden-brown on the outside and juicy and delicious on the inside. Serve directly from the instant crisp air fryer basket and enjoy while hot.

Nutrition: calories 291

Fat 23 g
Carbohydrates 3 g
Sugar 0 g
Protein 52 g
Cholesterol 165 mg

113) Tuscan pork chops

Preparation time: 10 minutes

cooking time: 10 minutes

total: 20 minutes   Servings: 4

Ingredients

1/4 cup all-purpose flour

1 teaspoon salt

3/4 teaspoons seasoned pepper

(1-inch-thick) boneless pork chops

1 tablespoon olive oil

3 to 4 garlic cloves

1/3 cup balsamic vinegar

1/3 cup chicken broth

3 plum tomatoes, seeded and diced

Tablespoons capers

Directions:

Preparing the ingredients. Combine flour, salt, and pepper press pork chops into flour mixture on both sides until evenly covered.

Air frying. Lock the air fryer lid. Cook in your instant crisp air fryer at 360 degrees for 14 minutes, flipping halfway through. While the pork chops cook, warm olive oil in a medium skillet. Add garlic and sauté for 1 minute; then mix in vinegar and chicken broth. Add capers and tomatoes and turn to high heat. Bring the sauce to a boil, stirring regularly, then add pork chops, cooking for one minute. Remove from heat and cover for about 5 minutes to allow the pork to absorb some of the sauce; serve hot.

Nutrition: calories 348

Fat 23 g

Carbohydrates 3 g

Sugar 0 g

Protein 52 g

Cholesterol 165 mg

114) Crispy breaded pork chops

Preparation time: 10 minutes

cooking time: 15 minutes

total: 25 minutes   Servings: 8

Ingredients

1/8 tsp. Pepper

¼ tsp. Chili powder

½ tsp. Onion powder

½ tsp. Garlic powder

1 ¼ tsp. Sweet paprika

2 tbsp. Grated parmesan cheese

1/3 c. Crushed cornflake crumbs

½ c. Panko breadcrumbs

1 beaten egg

Center-cut   boneless   pork   chops

Directions:

Preparing the ingredients. Ensure that your instant crisp air fryer is preheated to 400 degrees. Spray the basket with olive oil. With ½ teaspoon salt and pepper, season both sides of pork chops. Combine ¾ teaspoon salt with pepper, chili powder, onion powder, garlic powder, paprika, cornflake crumbs, panko breadcrumbs and parmesan cheese. Beat egg in another bowl. Dip pork chops into the egg and then crumb mixture. Add pork chops to instant crisp air fryer and spritz with olive oil.

Air frying. Close air fryer lid.

Set temperature to 400°f and set time to 12 minutes. Cook 12 minutes, making sure to flip over halfway through cooking process. Only add 3 chops in at a time and repeat the process with remaining pork chops.

Nutrition: calories 378

Fat 23 g
Carbohydrates 3 g
Sugar 0 g
Protein 52 g
Cholesterol 165 mg

115) Crispy roast garlic-salt pork

Preparation time: 5 minutes

cooking time: 45 minutes

total: 50 minutes   Servings: 4

Ingredients

1 teaspoon chinese five spice powder

1 teaspoon white pepper

2 pounds pork belly   2 teaspoons

   garlic salt

Directions:

Preparing the ingredients. Preheat the instant crisp air fryer to 390°f.

Mix all the spices in a bowl to create the dry rub.

Score the skin of the pork belly with a knife and season the entire pork with the spice rub.

Air frying. Place in the instant crisp air fryer basket, close air fryer lid and cook for 40 to 45 minutes until the skin is crispy.

Chop before serving.

Nutrition: calories 865

Fat 23 g
Carbohydrates 3 g
Sugar 0 g
Protein 52 g
Cholesterol 165 mg

116) Pork tenderloin and veggies

Preparation time: 5 minutes

Cooking time: 25 minutes   Smart points:

Servings: 4

Ingredients:

1-pound pork tenderloin, sliced
¼ cup cilantro, chopped
½ teaspoon garlic powder
1 tablespoon olive oil
1 green bell pepper, julienned
½ teaspoon chili powder   ½ teaspoon cumin, ground
Directions:

Heat up a pan that fits the air fryer with the oil over medium heat, add the pork and brown for 5 minutes.

Add the rest of the ingredients, toss, put the pan in the air fryer and cook at 400 degrees f for 20 minutes.

Divide between plates and serve.

Nutrition: calories 278

Fat 23 g

Carbohydrates 3 g

Sugar 0 g

Protein 52 g

Cholesterol 165 mg

117) Paprika pork mix

Preparation time: 5 minutes

Cooking time: 25 minutes   Smart

points:

Servings: 4

Ingredients:

1-pound pork stew meat, cubed

Teaspoons sweet paprika

A pinch of salt and black pepper

1 cup coconut cream

1 tablespoon butter, melted   1

tablespoon parsley, chopped

Directions:

Heat up a pan that fits the air fryer with the butter over medium heat, add the meat and brown for 5 minutes.

Add the remaining ingredients, toss, put the pan in the air fryer, cook at 390 degrees f for 20 minutes more, divide into bowls and serve.

Nutrition: calories 274 Fat 23 g

Carbohydrates 3 g

Sugar 0 g

Protein 52 g

Cholesterol 165 mg

118) Smoked pork chops

Preparation time: 5 minutes

Cooking time: 25 minutes   Smart

points:

Servings: 4

Ingredients:

Pork chops

1 tablespoon smoked paprika

1 tablespoon olive oil

Tablespoons balsamic vinegar

½ cup chicken stock   A pinch of salt and black pepper   Directions:

In a bowl, mix the pork chops with the rest of the ingredients and toss.

Put the pork chops in your air fryer's basket and cook at 390 degrees f for 25 minutes.

Divide between plates and serve.

Nutrition: calories 291

Fat 23 g

Carbohydrates 3 g

Sugar 0 g

Protein 52 g

Cholesterol 165 mg

119) Mustard pork chops

Preparation time: 5 minutes

Cooking time: 25 minutes   Smart

points:

Servings: 4

Ingredients:

Pork chops

A pinch of salt and black pepper

2/3 cup cream cheese, soft

¼ teaspoon garlic powder

Ounces beef stock

¼ teaspoon oregano, dried

1 tablespoon mustard

¼ teaspoon thyme, dried

1 tablespoon olive oil   1 tablespoon parsley, chopped

Directions:

In a baking dish that fits your air fryer, mix all the ingredients, introduce the pan in the fryer and cook at 400 degrees f for 25 minutes.

Divide everything between plates and serve.

Nutrition: calories 274

Fat 23 g

Carbohydrates 3 g

Sugar 0 g

Protein 52 g

Cholesterol 165 mg

120) Vinegar pork chops

Preparation time: 5 minutes

Cooking time: 25 minutes   Smart

points:

Servings: 4

Ingredients:

Tablespoons olive oil

Pork chops

A pinch of salt and black pepper

Garlic cloves, minced   Tablespoons cider vinegar

Directions:

Heat up a pan that fits the air fryer with the oil over medium-high heat, add the pork chops and brown for 5 minutes.

Add the rest of the ingredients, toss, put the pan in your air fryer and cook at 400 degrees f for 20 minutes.

Divide between plates and serve.

Nutrition:

calories 291 Fat

23 g

Carbohydrates 3 g

Sugar 0 g

Protein 52 g

Cholesterol 165 mg

121) Pork medallions   and garlic sauce

Preparation time: 5 minutes

Cooking time: 25 minutes   Smart

points:

Servings: 4

Ingredients:

1-pound pork tenderloin, sliced

A pinch of salt and black pepper

Tablespoons butter, melted

Teaspoons garlic, minced

1 teaspoon sweet paprika

Directions:

Heat up a pan that fits the air fryer with the butter over medium heat, add all the ingredients except the pork medallions, whisk well and simmer for 4-5 minutes.

Add the pork, toss, put the pan in your air fryer and cook at 380 degrees f for 20 minutes.

Divide between plates and serve with a side salad.

Nutrition: calories 275

Fat 23 g

Carbohydrates 3 g

Sugar 0 g

Protein 52 g

Cholesterol 165 mg

122) Coconut and chili pork

Preparation time: 5 minutes

Cooking time: 25 minutes   Smart

points:

Servings: 4

Ingredients:

Teaspoons chili paste

Garlic cloves, minced

Pork chops

1 shallot, chopped

1 and ½ cups coconut milk

Tablespoons olive oil

Tablespoons coconut amines   Salt and black pepper to the taste

Directions:

In a pan that fits your air fryer, mix the pork the rest of the ingredients, toss, introduce the pan in the fryer and cook at 400 degrees f for 25 minutes, shaking the fryer halfway.

Divide everything into bowls and serve.

Nutrition: calories 291

Fat 23 g

Carbohydrates 3 g

Sugar 0 g

Protein 52 g

Cholesterol 165 mg

123) Basil pork chops

Preparation time: 5 minutes

Cooking time: 25 minutes

Smart points:

Servings: 4

Ingredients:

Pork chops

A pinch of salt and black pepper

Teaspoons basil, dried

Tablespoons olive oil

½ teaspoon chili powder

Directions:

In a pan that fits your air fryer, mix all the ingredients, toss, introduce in the fryer and cook at 400 degrees f for 25 minutes.

Divide everything between plates and serve.

Nutrition: calories 291 Fat 23 g Carbohydrates 3 g

Sugar 0 g Protein 52 g Cholesterol 165 mg

124) Pork chops and tomato sauce

Preparation time: 5 minutes

Cooking time: 25 minutes Smart points:

Servings: 4

Ingredients:

1 tablespoon mustard

¼ cup tomato sauce

Pork chops

A pinch of salt and black pepper

1 teaspoon garlic powder

Teaspoons smoked paprika

1 and ½ teaspoons peppercorns, crushed

A pinch of cayenne pepper

A drizzle of olive oil

Directions:

Heat up a pan that fits your air fryer with the oil over medium heat, add the pork chops and brown for 5 minutes.

Add the rest of the ingredients, toss, put the pan in the fryer and cook at 400 degrees f for 20 minutes.

Divide everything between plates and serve.

Nutrition: calories 241

Fat 23 g
Carbohydrates 3 g
Sugar 0 g
Protein 52 g
Cholesterol 165 mg

125) Pork with lemon sauce

Preparation time: 15 minutes

Cooking time: 25 minutes   Smart

points:

Servings: 4

Ingredients:

Pork chops

Tablespoons olive oil

A pinch of salt and black pepper

Garlic cloves, minced

Teaspoons mustard

Teaspoons lemon zest, grated

Juice of 1 lemon

Directions:

In a bowl, mix the pork chops with the other ingredients, toss and keep in the fridge for 15 minutes

Put the pork chops in your air fryer's basket and cook at 390 degrees f for 25 minutes.

Divide between plates and serve with a side salad.

Nutrition: calories 263

Fat 23 g
Carbohydrates 3 g
Sugar 0 g
Protein 52 g
Cholesterol 165 mg

Cholesterol 165 mg

126) Pork roast

Preparation time: 5 minutes

Cooking time: 30 minutes

Smart points:

Servings: 4

Ingredients:

1-pound pork tenderloin, trimmed

A pinch of salt and black pepper

Tablespoons olive oil

Tablespoons   mustard

Tablespoons balsamic vinegar

Directions:

In a bowl, mix the pork tenderloin with the rest of the ingredients and rub well.

Put the roast in your air fryer's basket and cook at 380 degrees f for 30 minutes. Slice the roast, divide between plates and serve.

Nutrition: calories 241 Fat 23 g

Carbohydrates 3 g Sugar 0 g
Protein 52 g

127) Pork and green beans

Preparation time: 5 minutes

Cooking time: 25 minutes   Smart points:

Servings: 4

Ingredients:

Pork chops

Tablespoons coconut oil, melted

Garlic cloves, minced

A pinch of salt and black pepper

½ pound green beans, trimmed and halved   Tablespoons tomato sauce

Directions:

Heat up a pan that fits the air fryer with the oil over medium heat, add the pork chops and brown for 5 minutes.

Add the rest of the ingredients, put the pan in the machine and cook at 390 degrees f for 20 minutes.

Divide everything between plates and

serve

Nutrition: calories 284

Fat 23 g

Carbohydrates 3 g

Sugar 0 g

Protein 52 g

Cholesterol 165 mg

128) Greek pork and cheese

Preparation time: 5 minutes

Cooking time: 25 minutes   Smart

points:

Servings: 4

Ingredients:

Pounds pork tenderloin, cut into strips

Tablespoons coconut oil, melted

A pinch of salt and black pepper

Ounces baby spinach

1 cup cherry tomatoes, halved

1 cup feta cheese, crumbled

Directions:

Heat up a pan that fits your air fryer with the oil over medium high heat, add the pork and brown for 5 minutes.

Add the rest of the ingredients except the spinach and the cheese, put the pan to your air fryer, cook at 390 degrees f for 15 minutes.

Add the spinach, toss, and cook for 5 minutes more.

Divide between plates and serve with feta cheese sprinkled on top.

Nutrition: calories 286

Fat 23 g

Carbohydrates 3 g

Sugar 0 g

Protein 52 g

Cholesterol 165 mg

Fish

129) Lemon herb salmon

Preparation time: 10 minutes

Cooking time: 10 minutes

Servings: 2

Ingredients:

2 salmon fillets
2 tsp lime zest
2 tsp lemon zest
1 tbsp olive oil
1 tsp garlic, minced 1
tbsp thyme, diced
1 tbsp parsley, diced
Pepper
Salt
Directions:

In a small bowl, mix together lime zest, lemon zest, oil, garlic, thyme, parsley, pepper, and salt and rub over salmon.

Place the dehydrating tray in a multilevel air fryer basket and place basket in the instant pot.

Place salmon fillets on dehydrating tray.

Seal pot with air fryer lid and select air fry mode then set the temperature to 400 f and timer for 10 minutes.

Serve and enjoy.

Nutrition:

Calories 304
Fat 18.1 g
Carbohydrates 2.2 g
Sugar 0.2 g
Protein 34.9 g
Cholesterol 78 mg

130) Dijon crab cakes

Preparation time: 10 minutes

Cooking time: 14 minutes

Servings: 4

Ingredients:

1 egg, lightly beaten

1 lb. Crabmeat

1/2 cup crushed crackers

2 tsp worcestershire sauce

1 tsp dijon mustard

1 tsp dry mustard

1/3 cup mayonnaise

Directions:

Add all ingredients into the mixing bowl and mix until well combined.

Make four patties from mixture and place on a plate. Place patties in the refrigerator for 1 hour.

Place the dehydrating tray in a multilevel air fryer basket and place basket in the instant pot.

Place crab patties on dehydrating tray.

Seal pot with air fryer lid and select air fry mode then set the temperature to 350 f and timer for 14 minutes. Turn patties halfway through.

Serve and enjoy.

Nutrition:

Calories 222

Fat 9.2 g

Carbohydrates 24.5 g

Sugar 9.4 g

Protein 10.7 g

Cholesterol 69 mg

131) Pesto scallops

Preparation time: 10 minutes

Cooking time: 7 minutes

Servings: 4

Ingredients:

1 lb. Scallops

2 tsp garlic, minced

3 tbsp heavy cream

1/4 cup basil pesto

1 tbsp olive oil

Pepper

Salt

Directions:

Spray instant pot multi-level air fryer basket with cooking spray.

Season scallops with pepper and salt and adds into the air fryer basket and place basket into the instant pot.

Seal pot with air fryer lid and select air fry mode then set the temperature to 320 f and timer for 5 minutes. Turn scallops after 3 minutes.

Meanwhile, in a small saucepan, heat olive oil over medium heat. Add garlic and sauté for 30 seconds.

Add pesto and heavy cream and cook for 2 minutes. Remove from heat.

Add scallops into the mixing bowl. Pour pesto sauce over scallops and toss well.

Serve and enjoy.

Nutrition: Calories 171

Fat 8.5 g Carbohydrates 3.5 g
Sugar 0 g
Protein 19.4 g
Cholesterol 53 mg

132) Creamy parmesan shrimp

Preparation time: 10 minutes

Cooking time: 5 minutes

Servings: 4

Ingredients:

1 lb. Shrimp, deveined and cleaned
1 oz parmesan cheese, grated
1 tbsp garlic, minced
1 tbsp lemon juice
1/4 cup salad
dressing Directions:

Spray instant pot multi-level air fryer basket with cooking spray.

Add shrimp into the air fryer basket and place basket into the instant pot.

Seal pot with air fryer lid and select air fry mode then set the temperature to 400 f and timer for 5 minutes.

Transfer shrimp into the mixing bowl. Add remaining ingredients over shrimp and stir for 1 minute.

Serve and enjoy.

Nutrition:

Calories 219
Fat 8.4 g
Carbohydrates 6.3 g

Sugar 1 g

Protein 28.4 g

Cholesterol 248 mg

133) Delicious garlic butter salmon

Preparation time: 10 minutes

Cooking time: 7 minutes

Servings: 4

Ingredients:

1 lb. Salmon fillets

2 tbsp parsley, chopped

2 tbsp garlic, minced

1/4 cup parmesan cheese, grated

1/4 cup butter, melted

Pepper

Salt

Directions:

Season salmon with pepper and salt.

In a small bowl, mix together butter, cheese, garlic, and parsley and brush over salmon fillets.

Place the dehydrating tray in a multilevel air fryer basket and place basket in the instant pot.

Place salmon fillets on dehydrating tray.

Seal pot with air fryer lid and select air fry mode then set the temperature to 400 f and timer for 7 minutes.

Serve and enjoy.

Nutrition:

Calories 277

Fat 19.8 g

Carbohydrates 1.7 g

Sugar 0.1 g

Protein 24.3 g

Cholesterol 85 mg

134) Horseradish salmon

Preparation time: 10 minutes

Cooking time: 7 minutes

Servings: 2

Ingredients:

2 salmon fillets

1/4 cup breadcrumbs

2 tbsp olive oil

1 tbsp horseradish

Pepper

Salt

Directions:

Place the dehydrating tray in a multilevel air fryer basket and place basket in the instant pot.

Place salmon fillets on dehydrating tray.

In a small bowl, mix together breadcrumbs, oil, horseradish, pepper, and salt and spread over salmon fillets.

Seal pot with air fryer lid and select air fry mode then set the temperature to 400 f and timer for 7 minutes.

Serve and enjoy.

Nutrition:

Calories 413

Fat 25.8 g

Carbohydrates 10.6 g

Sugar 1.4 g

Protein 36.4 g

Cholesterol 78 mg

135) Pesto shrimp

Preparation time: 10 minutes

Cooking time: 5 minutes

Servings: 6

Ingredients:

1 lb. Shrimp, defrosted

14 oz basil pesto Directions:

Add shrimp and pesto into the mixing bowl and toss well.

Spray instant pot multi-level air fryer basket with cooking spray.

Add shrimp into the air fryer basket and place basket into the instant pot.

Seal pot with air fryer lid and select air fry mode then set the temperature to 400 f and timer for 5 minutes.

Serve and enjoy.

Nutrition:

Calories 105

Fat 1.7 g

Carbohydrates 2.9 g

Sugar 0.2 g

Protein 19.3 g

Cholesterol 159 mg

136) Delicious tilapia

Preparation time: 10 minutes

Cooking time: 8 minutes

Servings: 4

Ingredients:

2 tilapia fillets

1/4 tsp cayenne

1/2 tsp cumin

1 tsp garlic powder

1 tsp dried oregano

2 tsp brown sugar

2 tbsp paprika

Salt

Directions:

In a small bowl, mix together cayenne, cumin, garlic powder, oregano, sugar, paprika, and salt and rub over tilapia fillets.

Place the dehydrating tray in a multilevel air fryer basket and place basket in the instant pot.

Place tilapia fillets on dehydrating tray.

Seal pot with air fryer lid and select air fry mode then set the temperature to 400 f and timer for 8 minutes. Turn tilapia fillets halfway through.

Serve and enjoy.

Nutrition:

Calories 67

Fat 1.1 g

Carbohydrates 4.3 g

Sugar 2 g

Protein 11.2 g

Cholesterol 28 mg

137) Garlic butter shrimp

Preparation time: 10 minutes

Cooking time: 10 minutes

Servings: 4

Ingredients:

1 lb. Shrimp, peeled and deveined

2 tbsp olive oil

1/4 cup butter, melted

4 tbsp garlic, minced

Pepper

Salt

Directions:

Add shrimp into the mixing bowl. Add remaining ingredients and toss well.

Line instant pot multi-level air fryer basket with aluminum foil.

Add shrimp into the air fryer basket and place basket into the instant pot.

Seal pot with air fryer lid and select air fry mode then set the temperature to 400 f and timer for 10 minutes. Mix halfway through.

Serve and enjoy.

Nutrition:

Calories 309

Fat 20.5 g

Carbohydrates 4.5 g

Sugar 0.1 g

Protein 26.5 g

Cholesterol 269 mg

138) Crispy crust shrimp

Preparation time: 10 minutes

Cooking time: 20 minutes

Servings: 4

Ingredients:

1 lb. Shrimp, peeled and deveined

1 tsp garlic powder

1 tsp onion powder

1/2 cup breadcrumbs

2 eggs, lightly beaten

Pepper

Salt

Directions:

In a shallow bowl, whisk eggs with pepper and salt.

In a shallow dish, mix together breadcrumbs, onion powder, and garlic powder.

Place the dehydrating tray in a multilevel air fryer basket and place basket in the instant pot.

Dip shrimp in egg mixture then coat with breadcrumb and place on dehydrating tray.

Seal pot with air fryer lid and select air fry mode then set the temperature to 350 f and timer for 20 minutes. Turn shrimp halfway through.

Serve and enjoy.

Nutrition:

Calories 224

Fat 4.9 g

Carbohydrates 12.6 g

Sugar 1.4 g

Protein 30.6 g

Cholesterol 321 mg

139) Delicious crab cakes

Preparation time: 10 minutes

Cooking time: 15 minutes

Servings: 4

Ingredients:

1 egg, lightly beaten

1/2 cup breadcrumbs

1 cup crushed crackers

1 cup crab meat

2 tbsp parsley, chopped

1 tsp old bay seasoning

1 tsp worcestershire sauce

1/2 tsp dijon mustard

1 onion, chopped

2 tbsp mayonnaise

1/2 tsp salt Directions:

Add all ingredients into the mixing bowl and mix until well combined.

Make four patties from mixture and place on a plate. Place patties in the refrigerator for 1 hour.

Place the dehydrating tray in a multilevel air fryer basket and place basket in the instant pot.

Place crab patties on dehydrating tray.

Seal pot with air fryer lid and select air fry mode then set the temperature to 350 f and timer for 15 minutes. Turn patties halfway through.

Serve and enjoy.

Nutrition:

Calories 147

Fat 6 g

Carbohydrates 18.4 g

Sugar 3.6 g

Protein 5 g

Cholesterol 47 mg

140) Salmon patties

Preparation time: 10 minutes

Cooking time: 10 minutes

Servings: 4

Ingredients:

15 oz can salmon, drained and remove bones

1 tsp dill, chopped

1/2 cup breadcrumbs

1/4 cup onion, chopped

1 egg, lightly beaten

Pepper

Salt

Directions:

Add all ingredients into the mixing bowl and mix until well combined.

Make four patties from mixture and place on a plate.

Place the dehydrating tray in a multilevel air fryer basket and place basket in the instant pot.

Place salmon patties on dehydrating tray.

Seal pot with air fryer lid and select air fry mode then set the temperature to 370 f and timer for 10 minutes. Turn patties halfway through.

Serve and enjoy.

Nutrition:

Calories 220

Fat 8.3 g

Carbohydrates 10.6 g

Sugar 1.2 g

Protein 24.3 g

Cholesterol 99 mg

141) Honey mustard salmon

Preparation time: 10 minutes

Cooking time: 9 minutes

Servings: 2

Ingredients:

2 salmon fillets
2 tbsp dijon mustard
2 tbsp honey
1/4 cup mayonnaise
Pepper

Salt
Directions:

In a small bowl, mix together mustard, honey, mayonnaise, pepper, and salt and brush over salmon.

Place the dehydrating tray in a multilevel air fryer basket and place basket in the instant pot.

Place salmon fillets on dehydrating tray.

Seal pot with air fryer lid and select air fry mode then set the temperature to 350 f and timer for 9 minutes.

Serve and enjoy.

Nutrition:

Calories 424
Fat 21.4 g
Carbohydrates 25.2 g
Sugar 19.3 g
Protein 35.5 g
Cholesterol 86 mg

142) Classic tilapia

Preparation time: 10 minutes

Cooking time: 8 minutes

Servings: 2

Ingredients:

2 tilapia fillets
1 cup breadcrumbs
2 tbsp olive oil Directions:

Brush fish fillets with oil then coat with breadcrumbs.

Place the dehydrating tray in a multilevel air fryer basket and place basket in the instant pot.

Place coated fish fillets on dehydrating tray.

Seal pot with air fryer lid and select air fry mode then set the temperature to 370 f and timer for 8 minutes.

Serve and enjoy.

Nutrition:

Calories 426

Fat 17.9 g

Carbohydrates 38.9 g

Sugar 3.4 g

Protein 28.2 g

Cholesterol 55 mg

143) Coconut shrimp

Preparation time: 10 minutes

Cooking time: 6 minutes

Servings: 2

Ingredients:

1 egg, lightly beaten

1/2 lb. Shrimp, peeled

1/4 cup breadcrumbs

1/2 cup shredded coconut

1/4 cup flour

Pepper

Salt

Directions:

In one bowl, add flour. In the next bowl, whisk egg, pepper, and salt. In the third bowl, mix together coconut and breadcrumbs.

Line instant pot multi-level air fryer basket with aluminum foil.

Coat shrimp with flour then dip in egg then coat with coconut.

Place coated shrimp in the basket and place basket into the instant pot.

Seal pot with air fryer lid and select air fry mode then set the temperature to 400 f and timer for 6 minutes. Turn shrimp halfway through.

Serve and enjoy.

Nutrition:

Calories 347

Fat 11.7 g

Carbohydrates 26.6 g

Sugar 2.3 g

Protein 32.7 g

Cholesterol 321 mg

temperature to 400 f and timer for 10 minutes. Serve and enjoy.

Nutrition: Calories 288 Fat 16.8 g Carbohydrates 0.2 g Sugar 0.1 g Protein 34.7 g Cholesterol 94 mg

144) Garlic lemon salmon

Preparation time: 10 minutes

Cooking time: 10 minutes

Servings: 3

Ingredients:

3 salmon fillets

1/2 tsp dill, chopped

1/2 tbsp parsley, diced

1 tbsp lemon juice

1 1/2 tbsp butter, melted

1/2 tsp salt Directions:

In a small bowl, mix together butter, dill, parsley, lemon juice, and salt and brush over salmon fillets. Place the dehydrating tray in a multi-level air fryer basket and place basket in the instant pot. Place salmon fillets on dehydrating tray. Seal pot with air fryer lid and select air fry mode then set the

145) Coconut crusted fish fillets

Preparation time: 10 minutes

Cooking time: 8 minutes

Servings: 2

Ingredients:

2 tilapia fillets

1 egg, lightly beaten

1/4 cup coconut flour

1/2 cup flaked coconut

Salt

Directions:

In a shallow dish, mix together coconut flour, flaked coconut, and salt.

Dip fish fillets in egg then coat with coconut flour mixture.

Place the dehydrating tray in a multilevel air fryer basket and place basket in the instant pot.

Place coated fish fillets on dehydrating tray.

Seal pot with air fryer lid and select air fry mode then set the temperature to 400 f and timer for 8 minutes. Turn fish fillets halfway through.

Serve and enjoy.

Nutrition:

Calories 255

Fat 11.4 g

Carbohydrates 13.2 g

Sugar 1.4 g

Protein 26.5 g

Cholesterol 137 mg

146) Lemon garlic shrimp

Preparation time: 10 minutes

Cooking time: 5 minutes

Servings: 4

Ingredients:

1 lb. Shrimp

1 tbsp lemon juice

1/2 tbsp garlic powder

1/2 tbsp parsley, chopped

3 tbsp butter, melted

Pepper

Salt

Directions:

Add shrimp and remaining ingredients into the bowl and toss well.

Spray instant pot multi-level air fryer basket with cooking spray.

Add shrimp into the air fryer basket and place basket into the instant pot.

Seal pot with air fryer lid and select air fry mode then set the temperature to 400 f and timer for 5 minutes.

Serve and enjoy.

Nutrition:

Calories 216

Fat 10.6 g

Carbohydrates 2.6 g

Sugar 0.4 g

Protein 26.1 g

Cholesterol 262 mg

147) Tuna patties

Preparation time: 10 minutes

Cooking time: 6 minutes

Servings: 4

Ingredients:

1 egg, lightly beaten

1/4 cup breadcrumbs

1 tbsp mustard

Oz can tuna, drained

Pepper

Salt

Directions:

Add all ingredients into the mixing bowl and mix until well combined.

Make four patties from mixture and place on a plate.

Place the dehydrating tray in a multilevel air fryer basket and place basket in the instant pot.

Place tuna patties on dehydrating tray.

Seal pot with air fryer lid and select air fry mode then set the temperature to 400 f and timer for 6 minutes. Turn patties halfway through.

Serve and enjoy.

Nutrition:

Calories 113

Fat 2.7 g

Carbohydrates 5.9 g

Sugar 0.7 g

Protein 15.6 g

Cholesterol 56 mg

148) Fish with vegetables

Preparation time: 10 minutes

Cooking time: 25 minutes

Servings: 4

Ingredients:

1/2 lb. Cod fillet, cut into four pieces

1 cup cherry tomatoes

2 tbsp olive oil

1 cup baby potatoes, diced

Pepper

Salt

Directions:

Line instant pot multi-level air fryer basket with aluminum foil.

Toss potatoes with half olive oil and add into the air fryer basket and place basket into the instant pot.

Seal pot with air fryer lid and select bake mode then set the temperature to 380 f and timer for 15 minutes.

Add cod and cherry tomatoes in the basket.

Drizzle with remaining oil and season with pepper and salt.

Seal pot with air fryer lid and select bake mode then set the temperature to 380 f and timer for 10 minutes.

Serve and enjoy.

Nutrition:

Calories 146

Fat 7.7 g

Carbohydrates 8.8 g

Sugar 1.2 g

Protein 12 g

Cholesterol 28 mg

149) Tasty lemon tilapia

Preparation time: 10 minutes

Cooking time: 15 minutes

Servings: 2

Ingredients:

1/2 lb. Tilapia

1/2 tsp fresh lemon juice

1 tsp olive oil

1/2 lemon, sliced

1/2 tsp garlic powder

1/4 tsp dried thyme

1/4 tsp dried oregano

1/4 tsp pepper

1/2 tsp salt Directions:

Brush fish fillets with lemon juice and olive oil.

Mix together garlic powder, thyme, oregano, pepper, and salt and rub over fish fillets.

Place the dehydrating tray in a multilevel air fryer basket and place basket in the instant pot.

Place fish fillets on dehydrating tray. Place a lemon slice on top of fish fillets.

Seal pot with air fryer lid and select bake mode then set the temperature to 380 f and timer for 15 minutes.

Serve and enjoy.

Nutrition:

Calories 122

Fat 3.5 g

Carbohydrates 2.3 g

Sugar 0.6 g

Protein 21.4 g

Cholesterol 55 mg

150) Fish in garlic-chili sauce

Preparation time: 10 minutes

Cooking time: 15 minutes

Serving: 2

Ingredients:

Sauce

1/4 cup oyster sauce
1/4 cup soy sauce

To 10 cloves garlic, minced 1 tablespoon fish sauce
2 tablespoons brown sugar
1/4 teaspoon black pepper
1 tablespoon lime juice
3 red chilies, chopped
For the fish

2 whole red snappers
1 handful fresh coriander
1 handful fresh basil
4 tablespoon oil Directions:

Prepare the sauce by mixing all its ingredients: in a bowl.

Make a foil packet for each fish fillet and place a fillet in the pocket.

Place the fish pockets in the instant pot duo and top them with prepared sauce. Put on the air fryer lid and seal it.

Hit the "air fry button" and select 10 minutes of cooking time, then press "start."

Once the instant pot duo beeps, switch the instant pot to broil mode.

Broil the fish for 5 minutes in the pot.

Serve.

Nutrition:

Calories 265

Total fat 1.4g

Saturated fat 0.3g

Cholesterol 0mg Sodium 2952mg

Total carbohydrate 22.4g

Dietary fiber 0.7g

Total sugars 10g

Protein 3.5g

151) Halibut with mushroom sauce

Preparation time: 10 minutes

Cooking time: 26 minutes

Serving: 4

Ingredients:

4 halibut fillets

2 tablespoons butter   Salt to taste

Black pepper to taste

Sauce

3 tablespoons butter

4 to 6 oz. Mushrooms, sliced

4 to 6 green onions, trimmed, sliced

3 tablespoons flour

1/2 cup chicken broth

1 cup milk

1 tablespoon sherry

1/2 teaspoon seasoned salt   1/4 teaspoon garlic-seasoned pepper

Directions:

Mix melted butter with black pepper and salt in a small bowl.

Brush the halibut fillets with butter mixture then place them in the instant pot duo.

Put on the air fryer lid and seal it.

Hit the "bake button" at 350 degrees f and select 25 minutes of cooking time, then press "start."

Meanwhile, prepare the mushroom sauce and add butter to a saucepan.

Melt it then add mushrooms then sauté until golden brown.

Stir in green onion, then cook for 1 minute and stir in flour.

Slowly add milk, chicken broth, seasonings, and sherry, then stir cook until it thickens.

Once the instant pot duo beeps, remove its lid.

Transfer the halibut to the serving plate.

Top the halibut with mushroom sauce.

Serve.

Nutrition:

Calories 451

Total fat 14.1g

Saturated fat 5.4g

Cholesterol 113mg

Sodium 515mg

Total carbohydrate 9.7g

Dietary fiber 0.8g

Total sugars 3.7g

Protein 64.9g

152) Flounder with lemon butter

Preparation time: 10 minutes

Cooking time: 15 minutes

Serving: 4

Ingredients:

1 1/2 pounds flounder fillets, diced

1 teaspoon salt

1/8 teaspoon black pepper

4 tablespoons butter, melted

2 tablespoons lemon juice

2 teaspoons onion, minced

1 teaspoon paprika   Directions:

Spread the flounder pieces in a baking dish.

Drizzle salt and black pepper on top of the flounder.

Whisk melted butter with onion and lemon juice.

Pour this lemon-onion mixture over the fish along with paprika.

Place this pan in the instant pot duo.

Put on the air fryer lid and seal it.

Hit the "bake button" and select 15 minutes of cooking time, then press "start."

Once the instant pot duo beeps, remove its lid.

Serve.

Nutrition:

Calories 305

Total fat 14.3g

Saturated fat 8g

Cholesterol 146mg

Sodium 844mg

Total carbohydrate 0.7g

Dietary fiber 0.3g

Total sugars 0.3g

Protein 41.4g

153) Herbed sea bass

Preparation time: 10 minutes

Cooking time: 10 minutes

Serving: 4

Ingredients:

4 sea bass

1 1/2 to 2 bunches of parsley, finely chopped

Cloves of garlic, sliced

2 tablespoons of lemon juice

2 tablespoons of olive oil

Sea salt

1 tablespoon oregano

24 slices of tomato

Olive oil

1 cup white wine

3 cups of water

Directions:

Whisk lemon juice, parsley, garlic, oregano, salt, and olive oil in a bowl.

Add this parsley mixture inside the fish.

Pour water and wine into the instant pot duo.

Place the stuffed fish in the wine mixture and top it with tomato slices.

Put on the air fryer lid and seal it.

Hit the "bake button" and select 10 minutes of cooking time, then press "start."

Once the instant pot duo beeps, remove its lid.

Serve.

Nutrition:

Calories 198

Total fat 7.9g

Saturated fat 1.1g

Cholesterol 0mg

Sodium 9mg

Total carbohydrate 5.9g

Dietary fiber 1.8g

Total sugars 2.7g

Protein 27.3g

154) Quick coconut shrimp curry

Preparation time: 10 minutes

Cooking time: 1 minute

Servings: 2

Ingredients:

1 lb. Frozen shrimp

1/2 tsp curry powder

1/2 cup water

2 tbsp fresh cilantro, chopped

2 tbsp coconut milk

1 tbsp garam masala

1/8 tsp cayenne

1/2 tsp salt

Directions:

Add all ingredients into the instant pot except coconut milk and cilantro.

Stir well and seal the pot with a lid and cook on manual high pressure for 1 minute.

Once done then release pressure using the quick-release method than open the lid.

Stir in coconut milk. Garnish with cilantro and serve.

Nutrition:

calories 278

Fat 7.8 g

Carbohydrates 3.3 g

Sugar 0.5 g

Protein 46.8 g

Cholesterol 341 mg

155) Yummy fish tacos

Preparation time: 10 minutes

Cooking time: 8 minutes

Servings: 2

Ingredients:

2 tilapia fillets
1/4 cup fresh cilantro, chopped
2 tbsp lime juice

1 1/2 tbsp paprika
1 tsp olive oil
Pinch of salt   Directions:

Place fish fillets in the middle of parchment paper piece.

Drizzle fish fillet with oil and lime juice and season with paprika and salt.

Sprinkle cilantro on top of fish fillet.

Fold parchment paper around the fish fillet.

Pour 1 1/2 cups of water into the instant pot then place a trivet in the pot.

Place fish packet on top of the trivet.

Seal pot with lid and cook on manual high pressure for 8 minutes.

Once done then release pressure using the quick-release method than open the lid.

Serve and enjoy.

Nutrition:

calories 254

Fat 7.8 g

Carbohydrates

3.3 g

Sugar 0.5 g

Protein 46.8 g

Cholesterol 341 mg

156) Delicious scallops

Preparation time: 10 minutes

Cooking time: 2 minutes

Servings: 2

Ingredients:

1 lb. Scallops, thawed
2 1/2 tbsp maple syrup
1/2 cup coconut amines
1/4 tsp ground ginger
1/4 tsp garlic powder
1 tbsp olive oil
1/2 tsp sea salt   Directions:

Add oil into the instant pot and set the pot on sauté mode.

Add scallops to the pot and sear for 1 minute on each side.

In a small bowl, whisk together all remaining ingredients and pour over scallops.

Seal pot with lid and cook on steam mode for 2 minutes.

Once done then release pressure using the quick-release method than open the lid.

Serve and enjoy.

Nutrition:

calories 327

Fat 7.8 g

Carbohydrates 3.3 g

Sugar 0.5 g

Protein 46.8 g

Cholesterol 341 mg

157) Healthy shrimp rice

Preparation time: 10 minutes

Cooking time: 3 minutes

Servings: 2

Ingredients:

1 egg, lightly beaten

1/4 tsp ground ginger

1/8 tsp cayenne pepper

2 cups of water

1 small onion, chopped

1 1/2 tbsp soy sauce

1 1/2 tbsp olive oil

Oz frozen shrimp, peeled

1 cup rice, rinsed and drained

1 cup frozen carrots and peas

3 garlic cloves, minced

Pepper

Salt

Directions:

Add 1 tbsp oil in instant pot and set the pot on sauté mode.

Add egg into the pot and cook until scramble.

Transfer scrambled egg to a plate and set aside.

Add remaining oil, garlic, and onion and sauté for 2 minutes.

Add carrots, peas, shrimp, rice, water, ginger, soy sauce, pepper, and salt. Stir well.

Seal pot with lid and cook on manual high pressure for 5 minutes.

Once done then release pressure using the quick-release method than open the lid.

Add scrambled egg and stir well.

Serve and enjoy.

Nutrition:

calories 681

Fat 7.8 g

Carbohydrates 3.3 g

Sugar 0.5 g

Protein 46.8 g

Cholesterol 341 mg

158) Balsamic salmon

Preparation time: 10 minutes

Cooking time: 3 minutes

Servings: 2

Ingredients:

2 salmon fillets

1 cup of water

2 tbsp balsamic vinegar

1 1/2 tbsp honey

Pepper

Salt

Directions:

Season salmon with pepper and salt.

Mix together vinegar and honey.

Brush fish fillets with vinegar honey mixture.

Pour water into the instant pot then place trivet into the pot.

Place fish fillets on top of the trivet.

Seal pot with lid and cook on manual high pressure for 3 minutes.

Once done then release pressure using the quick-release method than open the lid.

Garnish with parsley and serve.

Nutrition:

calories 278

Fat 7.8 g

Carbohydrates 3.3 g

Sugar 0.5 g

Protein 46.8 g

Cholesterol 341 mg

159) Shrimp scampi

Preparation time: 10 minutes

Cooking time: 2 minutes

Servings: 2

Ingredients:

1 lb. Shrimp, peeled and deveined

1 cup of water

1/4 tsp red chili flakes

3 garlic cloves, minced

2 tbsp butter

2 tbsp lemon juice

Pepper

Salt

Directions:

Add butter into the instant pot and set the pot on sauté mode.

Add garlic, pepper, red chili flakes, and salt to the pot and sauté for 2 minutes. Add shrimp and water. Stir well.

Seal pot with lid and cook on manual high pressure for 2 minutes.

Once done then release pressure using the quick-release method than open the lid.

Stir in lemon juice and serve.

Nutrition:

calories

382

Fat 15.5 g

Carbohydrates 5.3 g

Sugar 0.4 g

Protein 52.2 g

cholesterol 508 mg

160) Dijon fish fillets

Preparation time: 10 minutes

Cooking time: 3 minutes

Servings: 2

Ingredients:

2 halibut fillets

1 tbsp dijon mustard

1 1/2 cups water

Pepper

Salt

Directions:

Pour water into the instant pot then place steamer basket in the pot.

Season fish fillets with pepper and salt and brush with dijon mustard.

Place fish fillets in the steamer basket.

Seal pot with lid and cook on manual high pressure for 3 minutes.

Once done then release pressure using the quick-release method than open the lid.

Serve and enjoy.

Nutrition:

calories 323

Fat 7 g

Carbohydrates 0.5 g

Sugar 0.1 g

Protein 60.9 g

Cholesterol 93 mg

161) Old bay seasoned haddock

Preparation time: 10 minutes

Cooking time: 7 minutes

Servings: 2

Ingredients:

1/2 lb. Haddock
1 tbsp fresh lemon juice
1/4 cup water
1 tbsp mayonnaise
1/4 tsp old bay seasoning
1/2 tsp olive oil

1/4 tsp dill, chopped   Directions:

Add water, mayonnaise, seasoning, olive oil, dill, and lemon juice in instant pot and stir well.

Place fish fillets in the pot.

Seal pot with lid and cook on manual high pressure for 7 minutes.

Once done then release pressure using the quick-release method than open the lid.

Serve and enjoy.

Nutrition:

calories 168

Fat 7 g

Carbohydrates 0.5 g

Sugar 0.1 g

Protein 60.9 g

Cholesterol 93 mg

162) Shrimp mac n cheese

Preparation time: 10 minutes

Cooking time: 10 minutes

Servings: 2

Ingredients:

1 1/4 cups elbow macaroni

1 tbsp butter

2/3 cup milk

1 bell pepper, chopped

15 shrimp

1 tbsp cajun spice

1/2 cup flour

1 cup cheddar cheese, shredded

Directions:

Add butter in instant pot and set the pot on sauté mode.

Add bell pepper and sauté for minutes.

Add water and pasta and stir well.

Seal pot with lid and cook on manual high pressure for 3 minutes.

Once done then release pressure using the quick-release method than open the lid.

Add cajun spices and flour and stir well.

Set pot on sauté mode. Add shrimp and cook for 2 minutes.

Add cheese and milk and stir well.

Serve and enjoy.

Nutrition:

calories 843

Fat 73 g

Carbohydrates 121.5 g

Sugar 4.1 g

Protein 126.9 g

Cholesterol 234 mg

163) Salmon rice pilaf

Preparation time: 10 minutes

Cooking time: 5 minutes

Servings: 2

Ingredients:

2 salmon fillets

1 cup chicken stock

1 tbsp butter

1/2 cup of rice

1/4 cup vegetable soup mix

1/4 tsp sea salt   Directions:

Add all ingredients except fish fillets into the instant pot and stir well.

Place steamer rack on top of rice mixture.

Place fish fillets on top of rack and season with pepper and salt.

Seal pot with lid and cook on manual high pressure for 5 minutes.

Once done then release pressure using the quick-release method than open the lid.

Serve and enjoy.

Nutrition: calories 274 Fat 7 g

Carbohydrates 0.5 g Sugar 0.1 g

Protein 60.9 g Cholesterol 93 mg

164) Perfect salmon dinner

Preparation time: 10 minutes

Cooking time: 2 minutes

Servings: 3

Ingredients:

1 lb. Salmon fillet, cut into three pieces
2 garlic cloves, minced
1/2 tsp ground cumin
1 tsp red chili powder
Pepper
Salt

Directions:

Pour 1 1/2 cups water into the instant pot then place trivet into the pot.

In a small bowl, mix together garlic, cumin, chili powder, pepper, and salt.

Rub salmon with spice mixture and place on top of the trivet.

Seal pot with lid and cook on steam mode for 2 minutes.

Once done then release pressure using the quick-release method than open the lid.

Serve and enjoy.

Nutrition:

calories 211

Fat 7 g

Carbohydrates 0.5 g

Sugar 0.1 g

Protein 60.9 g

Cholesterol 93 mg

165) Steam clams

Preparation time: 10 minutes

Cooking time: 3 minutes

Servings: 3

Ingredients:

1 lb. Mushy shell clams
2 tbsp butter, melted   1/4 cup
   white wine

1/2 tsp garlic powder

1/4   cup   fresh   lemon   juice

Directions:

Add white wine, lemon juice, garlic powder, and butter into the instant pot.

Place trivet into the pot.

Arrange clams on top of the trivet.

Seal pot with lid and cook on manual high pressure for 3 minutes.

Once done then allow   to release pressure naturally then open the lid.

Serve and enjoy.

Nutrition:

calories 336

Fat 7 g

Carbohydrates 0.5 g

Sugar 0.1 g

Protein 60.9 g

Cholesterol 93 mg

166) Mahi mahi fillets

Preparation time: 10 minutes

Cooking time: 13 minutes

Servings: 4

Ingredients:

Mahi-mahi fillets

29 oz can tomato, diced

1/2 onion, sliced

2 tbsp lemon juice

1/2 tsp dried oregano

3 tbsp butter

Pepper

Salt

Directions:

Add butter into the instant pot and set the pot on sauté mode.

Add onion and sauté for 2 minutes.

Add remaining ingredients except for fish fillets and sauté for 3 minutes.

Place fish fillets into the pot.

Seal pot with lid and cook on manual high pressure for 8 minutes.

Once done then release pressure using the quick-release method than open the lid.

Serve and enjoy.

Nutrition:

calories 323

Fat 7 g

Carbohydrates 0.5 g

Sugar 0.1 g

Protein 60.9 g

Cholesterol 93 mg

167) Easy garlic lemon shrimp

Preparation time: 10 minutes

Cooking time: 5 minutes

Servings: 3

Ingredients:

1 lb. Large shrimp

2 garlic cloves, minced

3 tbsp butter

1/2 tsp paprika

2 lemons, sliced

Directions:

Add butter into the pot and set the pot on sauté mode.

Add garlic and sauté for 1 minute.

Add shrimp, paprika, and lemon slices, and stirs well.

Seal pot with lid and cook on manual high pressure for 4 minutes.

Once done then allow   to release pressure naturally then open the lid.

Serve and enjoy.

Nutrition:

calories 229

Fat 7 g

Carbohydrates 0.5 g

Sugar 0.1 g

Protein 60.9 g

Cholesterol 93 mg

168) Cheesy tilapia

Preparation time: 10 minutes

Cooking time: 10 minutes

Servings: 2

Ingredients:

2 tilapia fillets

3/4 cup parmesan cheese, grated

2 tbsp fresh lemon juice

2 tbsp mayonnaise

Pepper

Salt

Directions:

In a bowl, mix together mayo, lemon juice, pepper, and salt and marinate fish fillets in this mixture.

Place marinated tilapia fillets into the instant pot.

Seal pot with lid and cook on manual high pressure for 7 minutes.

Once done then allow   to release pressure naturally then open the lid.

Top with cheese and cook on sauté mode for 3 minutes.

Serve and enjoy.

Nutrition:

calories 244

Fat 7 g

Carbohydrates 0.5 g

Sugar 0.1 g

Protein 60.9 g

Cholesterol 93 mg

169) Scallops curry

Preparation time: 10 minutes

Cooking time: 9 minutes

Servings: 4

Ingredients:

1 lb. Scallops

1 cup of coconut milk

1/2 tsp soy sauce

1/4 tsp nutmeg powder

1/2 cup red curry paste

1 1/2 cup chicken broth

1/2 tsp curry powder

1 tsp vinegar

1 tbsp olive oil

1/2 tsp salt

Directions:

Add oil into the instant pot and set the pot on sauté mode.

Add scallops and sauté for 3 minutes.

Add remaining ingredients and stir well.

Seal pot with lid and cook on manual high pressure for 6 minutes.

Once done then release pressure using the quick-release method than open the lid.

Serve and enjoy.

Nutrition:

calories 323

Fat 7 g

Carbohydrates 0.5 g

Sugar 0.1 g

Protein 60.9 g

Cholesterol 93 mg

170) Healthy shrimp boil

Preparation time: 10 minutes

Cooking time: 1 minute

Servings: 6

Ingredients:

2 lbs. Frozen shrimp, deveined

1 onion, chopped

1/2 tsp red pepper flakes

1 tbsp old bay seasoning

10 oz sausage, sliced

5 frozen half corn on the cobs

3 garlic cloves, crushed

1 cup chicken stock

1/2 tsp salt

Directions:

Add all ingredients into the instant pot and stir well.

Seal pot with lid and cook on manual high pressure for 1 minute.

Once done then release pressure using the quick-release method than open the lid.

Stir and serve.   1 lb. Shrimp, cooked   Nutrition: 1 cup asparagus, chopped   calories 408   1/2 onion, diced

Fat 7 g

Carbohydrates 0.5 g

Sugar 0.1 g

Protein 60.9 g

Cholesterol 93 mg

2 tsp olive oil

1/2 tsp pepper

 Salt

Directions:

   Add oil into the instant pot and set the pot on sauté mode.

   Add onion to the pot and sauté for 2-3 minutes.

171) Asparagus shrimp risotto

Preparation time: 10 minutes

Cooking time: 16 minutes

Servings: 6

Ingredients:

1 1/2 cups arborio rice

1 tbsp butter

3 1/2 cups chicken stock

1/2 cup white wine

1 cup mushrooms, sliced

1/4 cup parmesan cheese, grated

Nutrition:

calories 339 Fat

6.4 g

Carbohydrates 42.3 g

Sugar 1.6 g protein 23.3 g

Cholesterol 168 mg

Add mushrooms and cook for 5 minutes.

Add rice and cook until lightly brown.

Add stock and wine and stir well.

Seal pot with lid and cook on manual high pressure for 6 minutes,

Once done then release pressure using the quick-release method than open the lid.

Add asparagus and butter and cook on sauté mode for 1 minute.

Add shrimp and cook for 1 minute.

Stir in cheese and serve.

172) Basil tilapia

Preparation time: 10 minutes

Cooking time: 4 minutes

Servings: 4

Ingredients:

4 tilapia fillets

3 garlic cloves, minced

2 tomatoes, chopped

2 tbsp olive oil

1/2 cup basil, chopped

1/8 tsp pepper

1/4 tsp salt

Directions:

Pour half cup of water into the instant pot.

Add fish fillets into the steamer basket and season with pepper and salt.

Place a steamer basket into the pot.

Seal pot with lid and cook on manual high pressure for 2 minutes.

Once done then release pressure using the quick-release method than open the lid.

In a bowl, mix together tomatoes, basil, oil, garlic, pepper, and salt.

Place cooked fish fillets on serving plate and top with tomato mixture.

Serve and enjoy.

Nutrition: calories 168

Fat 6.4 g

Carbohydrates 42.3 g

Sugar 1.6 g protein 23.3 g

Cholesterol 168 mg

173) Delicious shrimp risotto

Preparation time: 10 minutes

Cooking time: 17 minutes

Servings: 4

Ingredients:

1 lb. Shrimp, peeled, deveined, and chopped

1 1/2 cups arborio rice

1/2 tbsp paprika

1/2 tbsp oregano, minced

1 red pepper, chopped

1 onion, chopped

1/2 cup parmesan cheese, grated

1 cup clam juice

3 cups chicken stock

1/4 cup dry sherry

2 tbsp butter

1/4 tsp pepper

1/2 tsp salt

Directions:

Add butter into the instant pot and set the pot on sauté mode.

Add onion and pepper and sauté until onion is softened.

Add paprika, oregano, pepper, and salt.

Stir for minute.

Add rice and stir for a minute.

Add sherry, clam juice, and stock. Stir well.

Seal pot with lid and cook on manual high pressure for 10 minutes.

Once done then release pressure using the quick-release method than open the lid.

Add shrimp and cook on sauté mode for 2 minutes.

Stir in cheese and serve.

Nutrition: calories 530

Fat 6.4 g

Carbohydrates 42.3 g

Sugar 1.6 g protein 23.3 g

Cholesterol 168 mg

174) Cajun shrimp

Preparation time: 10 minutes

Cooking time: 2 minutes

Servings: 4

Ingredients:

1 lb. Shrimp, peeled and deveined

15 asparagus spears

1 tbsp cajun seasoning

1 tsp olive oil Directions:

Pour 1 cup of water in instant pot then place the steam rack inside the pot.

Arrange asparagus on a steam rack in a layer.

Place shrimp on the top of asparagus.

Sprinkle cajun seasoning over shrimp and drizzle with olive oil.

Seal pot with lid and cook on steam mode for 2 minutes.

Once done then release pressure using the quick-release method than open the lid.

Serve and enjoy.

Nutrition:

calories

163

Fat 6.4 g

Carbohydrates 42.3 g

Sugar 1.6 g protein 23.3 g

Cholesterol 168 mg

175) Herb-lemon salmon packets

Preparation time: 15 min

Cooking time: 15 min

Servings: 4

Ingredients:

Dill weed, fresh, chopped (1 tablespoon)
Black pepper, ground (1/4 teaspoon)
Lemon slices, thin (4 pieces)
Butter, melted (4 tablespoons)
Salt (1/2 teaspoon)

Salmon fillets, skinless, 4-ounce (4 pieces)

Directions:

Preheat air fryer at 350 degrees fahrenheit.

Prepare 4 individual foil sheets. Mist with cooking spray.

Combine melted butter with pepper, salt, and dill weed. Toss with salmon. Fill each foil sheet with one fillet and half a slice of lemon. Twist and seal before placing on cookie sheet.

Air-fry for fifteen to twenty minutes.

Nutrition:

calories

265

Fat 6.4 g

Carbohydrates 42.3 g

Sugar 1.6 g protein 23.3 g

Cholesterol 168 mg

Seasoning, old bay (2 teaspoons) Shrimp, 15-count, cleaned, shell on (1/2 pound) Lemon, thinly sliced (1/2 piece)

Directions: Preheat air fryer at 350 degrees fahrenheit.

Toss all ingredients until well-mixed. Divide mixture among 2 foil sheets. Top each with lemon slices and cover with another foil. Twist and seal foil packs and add to a cookie sheet.

Air-fry for fifteen to twenty minutes.

Nutrition: calories 339 Fat 6.4 g

Carbohydrates 42.3 g Sugar 1.6 g protein 23.3 g Cholesterol 168 mg

176) Vegetables and shrimp packets

Preparation time: 5 min

Cooking time: 25 min

Servings: 2

Ingredients:

Vegetables, antioxidant blend, frozen (7 ounces)

177) Garlic butter shrimp packets

Preparation time: 10 min

Cooking time: 20 min

Servings: 4

Ingredients:

Olive oil (2 tablespoons)

Parsley, fresh, chopped (1 cup)
Shrimp, peeled, deveined, uncooked (1 pound)
Garlic cloves, grated (2 pieces)
Polenta, 1-pound, refrigerated, sliced into half-inch portions (1 roll) Salt (1/4 teaspoon)
Pepper (1/4 teaspoon)
Butter, melted (4 tablespoons)
Lemon juice (1 tablespoon)

For serving:

Lemon wedges
Parsley, fresh, chopped

Directions:

Preheat air fryer at 350 degrees fahrenheit.

Prepare 4 individual sheets of foil. Pull up sides to form into packets. Mist with cooking spray.
Fill each foil sheet with polenta slices, season with pepper and salt, and sprinkle with olive oil.
Toss shrimp with garlic, melted butter, lemon juice, and parsley.

Stir in pepper, red pepper flakes, and salt. Add shrimp mixture to foil sheets filled with polenta, including liquid.
Twist and seal foil packs and arrange on cookie sheet. Air-fry for fifteen to twenty minutes.

Nutrition: calories 340

Fat 6.4 g

Carbohydrates 42.3 g

Sugar 1.6 g protein 23.3 g

Cholesterol 168 mg

178) Lime-sake edamame and shrimp packets

Preparation time: 30 min

Cooking time: 20 min

Servings: 4

Ingredients:

Cilantro, fresh, chopped (1/4 cup)
Soy sauce (2 tablespoons) Shrimp, extra-large, peeled, deveined, uncooked (1 pound)
Sesame oil, toasted (1 tablespoon)

Green onions, w greens & whites separated, sliced thinly (4 pieces)

Sake (1/4 cup)

Honey (2 tablespoons)

Chili garlic sauce (1 tablespoon)

Edamame, shelled, frozen (10 ounces)

Lime wedges (8 pieces)

Directions:

Preheat air fryer at 350 degrees fahrenheit.

Prepare 4 individual sheets of foil. Pull up sides to form into packets. Mist with cooking spray.

Combine honey, chili garlic sauce, soy sauce, toasted sesame oil, and sake. Toss in shrimp, green onion whites, and frozen edamame.

Fill each foil sheet with mixture, then drizzle with juice from squeezed lime. Seal foil packs and arrange on cookie sheet.

Air-fry for fifteen to twenty minutes.

Open foil packs and serve topped with green onion greens, cilantro, and lime wedges.

Nutrition: calories 280

Fat 6.4 g

Carbohydrates 42.3 g

Sugar 1.6 g protein 23.3 g

Cholesterol 168 mg

179) Spicy lemon mini crab cakes

Preparation time: 40 min

Cooking time: 10 min

Servings: 24 Ingredients:

Crab cakes:

Green onions, sliced thinly, w greens & whites separated (2 pieces) Eggs, beaten (2 pieces)

Breadcrumbs, crispy, plain panko (1 cup)

Lump crabmeat, pasteurized,

refrigerated, cleaned (1 pound)

Mayonnaise (1/4 cup)

Chili garlic sauce (5 teaspoons)

Olive oil (2 tablespoons)

Dressing:

Lemon juice (1 tablespoon)

Garlic, minced (1 piece)

Mayonnaise (1/2

cup) Soy sauce (1

teaspoon)

Directions:
Preheat air fryer to

390 degrees

fahrenheit.

Mist cooking spray onto cookie sheet. Combine dressing ingredients, then cover and chill.

Stir together crabmeat, mayonnaise (1/4 cup), chili garlic sauce, breadcrumbs, eggs, and green onion whites. Mold mixture into 24 patties. Cover and chill for ten minutes.

Add patties to cookie sheet and brush all over with oil. Air-fry for ten to twelve minutes. Drain

before serving topped with sauce and green onion greens.

Nutrition: calories 100

Fat 6.4 g

Carbohydrates 42.3 g

Sugar 1.6 g protein 23.3 g

Cholesterol 168 mg

180) Fontina crab-filled mushrooms

Preparation time: 30 min

Cooking time: 25 min

Servings: 24 Ingredients:

Olive oil (1 tablespoon)

Lump crabmeat, fresh (4 ounces)

Lemon peel, grated (2 teaspoons)

Butter, melted (1 tablespoon)

Parmesan cheese, shredded (2 tablespoons)

Salt (1/4 teaspoon)

Baby belle mushrooms, washed, w stems removed (24 pieces) Breadcrumbs, crispy, plain panko (1/4 cup)

Fontina cheese, shredded (3/4 cup)

Green onions, chopped (2 tablespoons)

Seafood seasoning mix (1

teaspoon) Dill weed, fresh,

chopped (1 teaspoon)

Directions:

Preheat air fryer at 375 degrees fahrenheit. Mist cooking spray onto a pan.

Toss mushrooms caps in olive oil before adding to pan. Air-fry for twelve minutes.

Combine melted butter and breadcrumbs. Stir in fontina cheese, green onions, lemon peel, salt, parmesan cheese, dill weed, seasoning, and crabmeat. Stuff mushroom caps with filling, then air-fry for another ten to twelve minutes.

Nutrition: calories 40

Fat 2.5 g

Protein 2.0 g

Carbohydrates 2.0 g

181) Mediterranean shrimp skewers

Preparation time: 45 min

Cooking time: 10 min

Servings: 24   Ingredients:

Kalamata olives, pitted (24 pieces)
Lemon juice (2 tablespoons)
Olive oil (1 tablespoon)
Feta cheese, cubed (8 ounces)
Salt (1/2 teaspoon)
Cherry tomatoes (24 pieces)
Lemon peel, grated (1/2 teaspoon)
Red pepper, crushed (1/2 teaspoon)
Garlic cloves, minced (2 pieces)
Shrimp, large, peeled, deveined, w tail shells removed, uncooked (24 pieces)
Basil leaves, small (24 pieces) Cocktail skewers, 5-inch (24 pieces) Directions:

Preheat air fryer at 390 degrees fahrenheit.

Mist cooking spray onto a rimmed baking pan.

Combine lemon juice, salt, oil, lemon peel, red pepper, and garlic. Toss in shrimp.

Add shrimp mixture to pan and air-fry for ten to twelve minutes. Transfer to a bowl and chill for thirty minutes.

Alternately thread cherry tomatoes, basil leaves (folded in half), shrimp head ends, olives, shrimp tail ends, and feta cheese cubes onto skewers.

Serve and enjoy.

Nutrition: calories 45

Fat 3.0 g

Protein 3.0 g

Carbohydrates 1.0 g

182) Sesame shrimp flatbread

Preparation time: 15 min

Cooking time: 15 min

Servings: 10 Ingredients:

Cilantro leaves, fresh, chopped (1/4 cup)

Sesame oil, toasted (1 tablespoon)

Carrots, shredded (1 cup)

Soy sauce (1 tablespoon) Avocado, peeled, sliced thinly, sliced into thirds (1/2 piece)

Pizza crust, thin, refrigerated (11 ounces)

Shrimp, medium, peeled, deveined, w tail shells removed, uncooked (20 pieces)

Mozzarella cheese, shredded (2 cups)

Green onions, thinly sliced, w greens & whites separated (2 pieces)

Sriracha sauce (1 tablespoon) Directions:

Preheat air fryer to 375 degrees fahrenheit.

Mist cooking spray onto cookie sheet. Press unrolled dough onto sheet and coat with sesame oil. Air-fry for eight to ten minutes.

Toss shrimp with soy sauce.

Spread on top of crust the following: cheese (1 cup), carrots, green onion whites, shrimp mixture, and cheese (1 cup).

Air-fry for seven to eleven minutes. Serve topped with avocado, cilantro, and green onion greens, then drizzled with sriracha.

Nutrition: calories 200

Fat 9.0 g

Protein 11.0 g

Carbohydrates 18.0 g

183) Shrimp à la king

Preparation time: 15 min

Cooking time: 10 min

Servings: 6

Ingredients:

Skim milk (3/4 cup)

Biscuit mix (2¼cups 1 tablespoon)

Mixed vegetables, frozen (1 cup)

Pepper (1/8 teaspoon)

Clam chowder soup, prepared (18 ½ ounces)

Salad shrimp, cooked, frozen, thawed, rinsed (5 ounces) Dill weed, dried (1 teaspoon) Directions:

Preheat air fryer at 425 degrees fahrenheit.

Combine milk and biscuit mix (2 ¼ cups) to form a soft dough. Drop 6 tablespoons, one tablespoon at a time, onto cookie sheet. Air-fry for ten minutes.

Combine remaining ingredients in a saucepan and heat to boiling. Split each biscuit in half. Place each biscuit half on six individual plates, top with hot chowder mixture (1/4 cup), and cover with another biscuit half. Serve each filled biscuit topped with chowder mixture (1/4 cup).

Nutrition: calories 290

Fat 7.0 g

Protein 13.0 g

Carbohydrates 45.0 g

Beef

184) Cheeseburger egg rolls

Preparation time: 10

minutes cooking

time: 7 minutes

total: 17 minutes

Servings: 6

Ingredients

Egg roll wrappers

6 chopped dill pickle chips

1 tbsp. Yellow mustard

3 tbsp. Cream cheese

3 tbsp. Shredded cheddar cheese

½ c. Chopped onion

½ c. Chopped bell pepper

¼ tsp. Onion powder

¼ tsp. Garlic powder Ounces of raw lean ground beef

Directions:

In a skillet, add seasonings, beef, onion, and bell pepper. Stir and crumble beef till fully cooked, and vegetables are soft.

Take skillet off the heat and add cream cheese, mustard, and cheddar cheese, stirring till melted.

Pour beef mixture into a bowl and fold in pickles.

Lay out egg wrappers and place 1/6th of beef mixture into each one. Moisten egg roll wrapper edges with water. Fold sides to the middle and seal with water. Repeat with all other egg rolls.

Place rolls into air fryer, one batch at a time.

Pour into the oven rack/basket. Place the rack on the middle-shelf of the air fryer oven. Set temperature to 392°f and set time to 7 minutes.

Nutrition: calories 163 Fat 9.0 g

Protein 11.0 g Carbohydrates 18.0 g

185) Air fried grilled steak

Preparation time: 5

minutes cooking

time: 45 minutes

total: 50 minutes

Servings: 2

Ingredients

2 top sirloin steaks

3 tablespoons butter, melted

3 tablespoons olive

oil Salt and

pepper to taste

Directions:

Preheat the air fryer oven for 5 minutes.

Season the sirloin steaks with olive oil, salt and pepper.

Place the beef in the air fryer basket.

Cook for 45 minutes at 350°f.

Once cooked, serve with butter.

Nutrition: calories 241 Fat 30.0 g

Protein 53.0 g Carbohydrates 18.0 g

186) Juicy cheeseburgers

Preparation time: 5 minutes

cooking time: 15 minutes

total: 20 minutes Servings: 4

Ingredients

1 pound 93% lean ground beef

1 teaspoon worcestershire sauce

1 tablespoon burger seasoning

Salt

Pepper

Cooking oil

4 slices cheese

Buns

Directions:

In a large bowl, mix the ground beef, worcestershire, burger seasoning, and salt and pepper to taste until well blended. Spray the air fryer basket with cooking oil. You will need only a quick spritz. The burgers will produce oil as they cook. Shape the mixture into 4 patties. Place the burgers in the air fryer. The burgers should fit without the need to stack, but stacking is okay if necessary.

Pour into the oven rack/basket. Place the rack on the middle-shelf of the air fryer oven. Set temperature to 375°f and set time to 8 minutes. Cook for 8 minutes. Open the air fryer and flip the burgers. Cook for an additional 3 to 4 minutes. Check the inside of the burgers to determine if they have finished cooking. You can stick a knife or fork in the center to examine the color.

Top each burger with a slice of cheese. Cook for an additional minute, or until the cheese has melted. Serve on buns with any additional toppings of your choice.

Nutrition: calories 241

Fat 30.0 g

Protein 53.0 g

Carbohydrates 18.0 g

187) Spicy thai beef stir-fry

Preparation time: 15 minutes

cooking time: 9 minutes   total:

24 minutes Servings: 4

Ingredients

1-pound sirloin steaks, thinly sliced

2 tablespoons lime juice, divided

⅓ cup crunchy peanut butter

½ cup beef broth

1 tablespoon olive oil

1½ cups broccoli florets

2 cloves garlic, sliced 1 to 2

red chili peppers, sliced

Directions:

In a medium bowl, combine the steak with 1 tablespoon of the lime juice. Set aside.

Combine the peanut butter and beef broth in a small bowl and mix well.

Drain the beef and add the juice from the bowl into the peanut butter mixture.

In a 6-inch metal bowl, combine the olive oil, steak, and broccoli.

Pour into the oven rack/basket. Place the rack on the middle-shelf of the air fryer oven. Set temperature to 375°f and set time to 4 minutes. Cook for 3 to 4 minutes or until the steak is almost cooked and the broccoli is crisp and tender, shaking the basket once during cooking time.

Add the garlic, chili peppers, and the peanut butter mixture and stir.

Cook for 3 to 5 minutes or until the sauce is bubbling and the broccoli is tender.

Serve over hot rice.

Nutrition: calories 387

Fat 30.0 g

Protein 53.0 g

Carbohydrates 18.0 g

188) Beef brisket recipe from texas

Preparation time: 15 minutes   cooking time: 1hour and 30 minutes

Servings: 8

Ingredients

1 ½ cup beef stock

1 bay leaf

1 tablespoon garlic powder

1 tablespoon onion powder

2 pounds beef brisket, trimmed

2 tablespoons chili powder

2 teaspoons dry mustard

4 tablespoons olive

oil   Salt   and

pepper to taste

Directions:

Preheat the air fryer oven for 5 minutes. Place all ingredients in a deep baking dish that will fit in the air fryer.

Bake for 1 hour and 30 minutes at 400°f.

Stir the beef every after 30 minutes to soak in the sauce.

Nutrition: calories 312

Fat 30.0 g

Protein 53.0 g

Carbohydrates 18.0 g

189) Copycat taco bell crunch wraps

Preparation time: 10 minutes

cooking time: 2 minutes   total:

15 minutes Servings: 6

Ingredients

6 wheat tostadas

2 c. Sour cream

2 c. Mexican blend cheese

2 c. Shredded lettuce

12 ounces low-sodium nacho cheese

3 roma tomatoes

6 12-inch wheat tortillas

1 1/3 c. Water

2 packets low-sodium taco seasoning

2 pounds of lean ground beef

Directions:

Ensure your air fryer is preheated to 400 degrees.

Make beef according to taco seasoning packets.

Place 2/3 c. Preparation red beef, 4 tbsp. Cheese, 1 tostada, 1/3 c. Sour cream, 1/3 c. Lettuce, 1/6th of tomatoes and 1/3 c. Cheese on each tortilla.

Fold up tortillas edges and repeat with remaining ingredients.

190) Steak and mushroom gravy

Preparation time: 15 minutes

pinch cooking time: 15 minutes of salt and pepper.
 total: 30 minutes

Servings: 4

Ingredients cayenne, and onion powder.
4 cubed steaks

2 large eggs

1/2 dozen mushrooms

4 tablespoons unsalted butter

4 tablespoons black pepper

Lay the folded sides of tortillas down into the air fryer and spray with olive oil.

Set temperature to 400°f and set time to 2 minutes. Cook 2 minutes till browned.

Nutrition: calories 311 Fat 30.0 g

Protein 53.0 g Carbohydrates 18.0 g

Directions:

Mix 1/2 flour and a pinch of black pepper in a shallow bowl or on a plate.

Beat 2 eggs in a bowl and mix in a

In another shallow bowl mix together the other half of the flour with a pepper to taste, garlic powder, paprika,

Chop mushrooms and set aside.

Press your steak into the first flour bowl,

then dip in egg, then press the steak into

the second-floor bowl until covered completely.

182

2 tablespoons salt

1/2 teaspoon onion powder

1/2 teaspoon garlic powder

1/4 teaspoon cayenne powder

1 1/4 teaspoons paprika

to sauté.

1/3 cup flour

Tablespoons vegetable oil

Mix in whole milk and simmer.

Serve over steak for breakfast, lunch, or dinner.

Nutrition: calories 442

Fat 30.0 g

Protein 53.0 g

Carbohydrates 18.0 g

Pour into the oven rack/basket. Place

the rack on the middle-shelf of the air fryer oven. Set temperature to 360°f and set time to 15 minutes flipping halfway

through.

While the steak cooks, warm the butter over medium heat and add mushrooms 1 1/2 cups whole milk

Add 4 tablespoons of the flour and pepper mix to the pan and mix until there are no clumps of flour.

Preparation time: 5

minutes   cooking time: 30

minutes   total: 35 minutes

Servings: 4

Ingredients

1 green bell pepper, seeded and chopped

1 onion, chopped

1-pound ground beef

3 cloves of garlic, minced

3 tablespoons olive oil

191) Air fryer beef casserole

6 cups eggs, beaten Salt

and pepper to taste

Directions:

Preheat the air fryer oven for 5 minutes.

In a baking dish that will fit in the air fryer, mix the ground beef, onion, garlic, olive oil, and bell pepper. Season with salt and pepper to taste.

Pour in the beaten eggs and give a good stir.

Place the dish with the beef and egg mixture in the air fryer.

Pour into the oven rack/basket. Place the rack on the middle-shelf of the air fryer oven. Set temperature to 325°f and set time to 30 minutes. Bake for 30 minutes.

Nutrition: calories 241

Fat 30.0 g

Protein 53.0 g

Carbohydrates 18.0 g

192) Meat lovers' pizza

Preparation time: 10 minutes

cooking time: 12 minutes

total: 22 minutes Servings: 2

Ingredients

1   pre-preparation red 7-inch pizza pie crust defrosted if necessary.

1/3 cup of marinara sauce.

2   ounces of grilled steak, sliced into bitesized pieces

2 ounces of salami, sliced fine

2 ounces of pepperoni, sliced fine

¼ cup of american cheese ¼ cup of

shredded mozzarella cheese

Directions:

Preheat the air fryer oven to 350 degrees. Lay the pizza dough flat on a sheet of parchment paper or tin foil, cut large enough to hold the entire pie crust, but small enough that it will leave the edges of the air frying basket uncovered to allow for air circulation. Using a fork, stab the pizza dough several times across the surface – piercing the pie crust will allow air to circulate throughout the crust and ensure even cooking. With a deep soup spoon, ladle the marinara sauce onto the pizza dough, and spread evenly in expanding circles over the surface of the piecrust. Be sure to leave at least ½ inch of bare dough around the edges, to ensure that extra-crispy crunchy first bite of the crust! Distribute the pieces of steak and the slices of salami and pepperoni evenly over the sauce-covered dough, then sprinkle the cheese in an even layer on top.

Set the air fryer timer to 12 minutes and place the pizza with foil or paper on the fryer's basket surface. Again, be sure to leave the edges of the basket uncovered to allow for proper air circulation, and don't let your bare fingers touch the hot surface. After 12 minutes, when the air fryer oven shuts off, the cheese should be perfectly melted and lightly crisped, and the pie crust should be golden brown. Using a spatula – or two, if necessary, remove the pizza from the air fryer basket and set on a serving plate. Wait a few minutes until the pie is cool enough to handle, then cut into slices and serve.

Nutrition: calories 256

Fat 30.0 g

Protein 53.0 g

Carbohydrates 18.0 g

193) Chimichurri skirt steak

Preparation time: 10 minutes

cooking time: 8 minutes

total: 18 minutes Servings: 2

Ingredients

2 x 8 oz skirt steak

1 cup finely chopped parsley

¼ cup finely chopped mint

2 tbsp fresh oregano (washed & finely chopped)

3 finely chopped cloves of garlic

1 tsp red pepper flakes (crushed)

1 tbsp ground cumin

1 tsp cayenne pepper

2 tsp smoked paprika

1 tsp salt

¼ tsp pepper

¾ cup oil

3 tbsp red wine vinegar

Directions:

Throw all the ingredients in a bowl (besides the steak) and mix well.

Put ¼ cup of the mixture in a plastic baggie with the steak and leave in the fridge overnight (2–24hrs).

Leave the bag out at room temperature for at least 30 min before popping into the air fryer. Preheat for a minute or two to 390° f before cooking until med–rare (8–10 min). Pour into the oven rack/basket. Place the rack on the middle-shelf of the air fryer oven. Set temperature to 390°f and set time to 10 minutes.

Put 2 tbsp of the chimichurri mix on top of each steak before serving.

Nutrition: calories 502

Fat 30.0 g

Protein 53.0 g

Carbohydrates 18.0 g

194) Country fried steak

Preparation time: 5 minutes

cooking time: 12 minutes

total: 20 minutes Servings:

2

Ingredients

1 tsp. Pepper

2 c. Almond milk

2 tbsp. Almond flour

6 ounces ground sausage meat

1 tsp. Pepper

1 tsp. Salt

1 tsp. Garlic powder

1 tsp. Onion powder

1 c. Panko breadcrumbs

1 c. Almond flour

3 beaten eggs

6 ounces sirloin steak, pounded till thin

Directions:

Season panko breadcrumbs with spices. Dredge steak in flour, then egg, and then seasoned panko mixture.
Place into air fryer basket.

Set temperature to 370°f and set time to 12 minutes.

To make sausage gravy, cook sausage and drain off fat, but reserve 2 tablespoons.

Add flour to sausage and mix until incorporated. Gradually mix in milk over medium to high heat till it becomes thick.

Season mixture with pepper and cook 3 minutes longer.

Serve steak topped with gravy and enjoy.

Nutrition: calories 395

Fat 30.0 g

Protein 53.0 g

Carbohydrates 18.0 g

195) Creamy burger & potato bake

Preparation time: 5

minutes   cooking time: 55

minutes   total: 60 minutes

Servings: 3

Ingredients

Salt to taste

Freshly ground pepper, to taste

1/2 (10.75 ounce) can condensed cream of mushroom soup

1/2-pound lean ground beef

1-1/2 cups peeled and thinly sliced potatoes

1/2 cup shredded cheddar cheese

1/4 cup chopped onion   1/4 cup

and 2 tablespoons milk

Directions:

Lightly grease baking pan of air fryer with cooking spray. Add ground beef. For 10 minutes, cook on 360°f. Stir and crumble halfway through cooking time.

Meanwhile, in a bowl, whisk well pepper, salt, milk, onion, and mushroom soup. Mix well.

Drain fat off ground beef and transfer beef to a plate.

In same air fryer baking pan, layer ½ of potatoes on bottom, then ½ of soup mixture, and then ½ of beef. Repeat process. Cover pan with foil.

Cook for 30 minutes. Remove foil and cook for another 15 minutes or until potatoes are tender. Serve and enjoy. Nutrition: calories 399 Fat 26.0 g

Protein 43.0 g Carbohydrates 18.0 g

196) Beefy 'n cheesy spanish rice casserole

Preparation time: 10 minutes

cooking time: 50 minutes

total: 60 minutes Servings: 3

Ingredients

2 tablespoons chopped green bell pepper

1 tablespoon chopped fresh cilantro

1/2-pound lean ground beef

1/2 cup water

1/2 teaspoon salt

1/2 teaspoon brown sugar

1/2 pinch ground black pepper

1/3 cup uncooked long grain rice

1/4 cup finely chopped onion

1/4 cup chili sauce

1/4 teaspoon ground cumin

1/4 teaspoon worcestershire sauce

1/4 cup shredded cheddar cheese 1/2

(14.5 ounce) can canned tomatoes

Directions:

Lightly grease baking pan of air fryer with cooking spray. Add ground beef.

For 10 minutes, cook on 360°f. Halfway through cooking time, stir and crumble beef. Discard excess fat,

Stir in pepper, worcestershire sauce, cumin, brown sugar, salt, chili sauce, rice, water, tomatoes, green bell pepper, and onion. Mix well. Cover pan with foil and cook for 25 minutes. Stirring occasionally.

Give it one last good stir, press down firmly and sprinkle cheese on top.

Cook uncovered for 15 minutes at 390°f until tops are lightly browned.

Serve and enjoy with chopped cilantro.

Nutrition: calories 241

Fat 30.0 g

Protein 53.0 g

Carbohydrates 18.0 g

197) Warming winter   beef with celery

Preparation time: 5 minutes

cooking time: 12 minutes

total: 15 minutes Servings:

4

Ingredients

Ounces tender beef, chopped

1/2 cup leeks, chopped

1/2 cup celery stalks, chopped

2 cloves garlic, smashed

2 tablespoons red cooking wine

3/4 cup cream of celery soup

2 sprigs rosemary, chopped

1/4 teaspoon smoked paprika

3/4 teaspoons salt

1/4 teaspoon black pepper, or to taste

Directions:

Add the beef, leeks, celery, and garlic to the baking dish; cook for about 5 minutes at 390 degrees f.

Once the meat is starting to tender, pour in the wine and soup. Season with rosemary, smoked paprika, salt, and black pepper. Now, cook an additional 7 minutes.

Nutrition: calories 255

Fat 30.0 g

Protein 53.0 g

Carbohydrates 18.0 g

198) Beef & veggie spring rolls

Preparation time: 5 minutes

cooking time: 12 minutes

total: 55 minutes   Servings:

10

Ingredients

2-ounce asian rice noodles

1 tablespoon sesame oil

7-ounce ground beef

1 small onion, chopped

3 garlic cloves, crushed

1 cup fresh mixed vegetables

1 teaspoon soy sauce

1 packet spring roll skins

2 tablespoons water Olive oil, as

  required

Directions:

Soak the noodles in warm water till soft.

Drain and cut into small lengths. In a pan heat the oil and add the onion and garlic and sauté for about 4-5 minutes.

Add beef and cook for about 4-5 minutes.

Add vegetables and cook for about 5-7 minutes or till cooked through.

Stir in soy sauce and remove from the heat.

Immediately, stir in the noodles and keep aside till all the juices have been absorbed.

Preheat the air fryer oven to 350 degrees

f.

Place the spring rolls skin onto a smooth surface.

Add a line of the filling diagonally across.

Fold the top point over the filling and then fold in both sides.

On the final point brush, it with water before rolling to seal.

Brush the spring rolls with oil.

Arrange the rolls in batches in the air fryer and cook for about 8 minutes.

Repeat with remaining rolls. Now, place spring rolls onto a baking sheet.

Bake for about 6 minutes per side.

Nutrition: calories 265

Fat 30.0 g

Protein 53.0 g

Carbohydrates 18.0 g

199) Easy beef bourguignon kabobs

Preparation time: 45 mins

Cooking time: 10 mins

Servings: 4

Ingredients:

Thyme leaves, fresh, chopped (1 teaspoon)
Red wine vinegar (1 tablespoon
Butter, melted (2 tablespoons)
Yellow onion, medium, sliced into wedged chunks (1 piece)
Parsley leaves, fresh, chopped (1 tablespoon)
Olive oil (2 tablespoons)
Salt (1 ¼ teaspoons)
Bacon slices, thick cut, 2-inch (12 pieces)
Honey (1 tablespoon)
Red wine, dry (1/2 cup)
Garlic cloves, minced (2 pieces)
Mushrooms, fresh, halved (1/2 pound)
Beef steak, top sirloin, boneless, cubed (1 ½ pounds)
Sage leaves, fresh, chopped (1 teaspoon)
Skewers, bamboo, 10-inch (8 pieces)
Directions:

Preheat air fryer at 390 degrees fahrenheit.

Combine olive oil with honey and vinegar.

Toss onion wedges and mushrooms with a mixture of melted butter, salt, wine, and garlic. Alternately thread onion and mushrooms onto 4 skewers.

Coat beef with remaining wine mixture, then alternately thread with bacon on other 4 skewers.

Air-fry for ten to twelve minutes. Serve sprinkled with sage, thyme, and parsley.

Nutrition: calories 241

Fat 30.0 g

Protein 53.0 g

Carbohydrates 18.0 g

200) Double decker tacos

Preparation time: 15 min

Cooking time: 5 min

Servings: 6

Ingredients:

Chicken/beef (2 cups)
Taco shells, hard (6 pieces)

Tortillas, soft (6 pieces)
Refried beans, heated (1 can)
Toppings: salsa, sour cream, diced avocado, cheese, etc.

Directions:

Preheat air fryer to 325 degrees fahrenheit.

Spread the top of each tortilla with refried beans (2 tablespoons) and then wrap around a taco shell.

Mist cooking spray onto filled taco shells and tortillas. Air-fry for five minutes, turning halfway.

Serve and enjoy.

Nutrition: calories 290 Fat 30.0 g

Protein 53.0 g Carbohydrates 18.0 g

201) Tasty taco cupcakes

Nutrition: calories 270 fat 9.0 g protein 12.0 g carbohydrates 35.0 g

Preparation time: 10 min cooking time: 20 min Servings:

18

Ingredients:

Wonton wrappers (36 pieces)

Taco seasoning mix (1 ounce)

Tortilla chips (36 pieces)

Ground beef (1 pound)

Water (2/3 cup)

Refried beans (16 ounces)

Cheddar cheese, shredded (2 cups)

Toppings: cilantro, sour cream, onion, diced tomatoes Directions:

Preheat air fryer to 350 degrees fahrenheit. Mist cooking spray onto 18 muffin cups.

Cook beef in skillet until browned; drain fat before adding water and taco seasoning mix. Let simmer for four to five minutes.

Fill each muffin cup with a wonton wrapper. Fill each wrapper with refried beans (1 tablespoon), then top with crushed tortilla chip (1 piece), taco meat (1 tablespoon), and shredded cheese (1 tablespoon).

Air-fry for fifteen to eighteen minutes. Serve topped with desired toppings.

Nutrition: calories 251

Fat 30.0 g

Protein 53.0 g

Carbohydrates 18.0 g

202) Mouthwatering lasagna cupcakes

Preparation time: 15 min

Cooking time: 20 min

Servings: 12

Ingredients:

Ricotta cheese (3/4 cup)

Parmesan cheese, grated (1 ¾ cups)

Pasta sauce, muir glen (1 cup)

Ground beef (1/3 pound)

Wonton wrappers (24 pieces)

Mozzarella cheese, shredded (1 ¾ cups)

Basil Salt Pepper Directions:

Preheat air fryer to 350 degrees fahrenheit. Mist cooking spray onto a muffin tin.

Cook beef in skillet until browned, then sprinkle with pepper and salt before draining.

25

Cut 2 ¼-inch-wide circles out of wonton wrappers.

Set aside ¾ cup each of mozzarella cheese and parmesan cheese.

Press a wonton wrapper into each muffin cup. Top each with layered parmesan, ricotta, and mozzarella cheeses, then with meat mixed with pasta sauce. Finish each by topping with reserved parmesan cheese and mozzarella cheese.

Air-fry for eighteen to twenty minutes. Let cool before serving garnished with basil.

Nutrition: calories 241 Fat 30.0 g

Protein 53.0 g Carbohydrates 18.0 g

203) Cheeseburger minis

Preparation time: 20 min

Cooking time: 25 min

Servings: 9

Ingredients:

Dill pickle, diced (1 piece)
White onion, diced (1/2 piece)
Salt (1/4 teaspoon)
Pepper (1/4 teaspoon)
Roma tomatoes, diced (2 pieces)
Ground beef, lean (1 pound) Pizza crust, classic, refrigerated (1 container)
Cheddar cheese, grated (4 ounces)
Butter
Mustard
Ketchup

Directions:

Preheat air fryer to 350 degrees fahrenheit.

Cook onions in oil until softened. Stir in ground beef and cook until browned and broken up. Season with pepper and salt. Set aside.

Grease a muffin tin with cooking spray before filling with 9 dough sheets (cut out from lightly rolled out pizza crust), pressing down to create crusts. Fill each crust with beef mixture, then air-fry for sixteen to eighteen minutes. Sprinkle with cheese and air-fry for another two to three minutes.

Serve garnished with desired toppings.

Nutrition: calories 290

Fat 30.0 g

Protein 53.0 g

Carbohydrates 18.0 g

204) Friese salami salad

Preparation time: 10 min

Cooking time: 30 min

Servings: 8

Ingredients:

Friese, torn (4 bunches) Beef salami slices, kosher, sliced into quarter-inch strips (6 ounces)

Mustard, coarse grained (2 teaspoons)

Garlic clove, minced (1 piece)

Black pepper, coarsely ground (1/4 teaspoon)

Olive oil, extra virgin (1/4 cup)

Red onion, medium, sliced (1/2 piece)

Sherry vinegar (1 tablespoon 1/3 cup)

Kosher salt (1/2 teaspoon)

Grape tomatoes, halved (1 pint)

Directions:

Preheat air fryer at 350 degrees fahrenheit.

Brush salami strips with oil. Place in baking pan and air-fry for fifteen minutes.

Stir garlic and onion in same pan and air-fry for ten minutes. Stir in salt, mustard, pepper, and vinegar, and airfry for five minutes.

Toss tomatoes and fries with vinegar mixture, then sprinkle on top with salami strips.

Serve and enjoy.

Nutrition: calories 120 Fat 30.0 g

Protein 53.0 g

Carbohydrates 18.0 g

205) Easy tortilla casserole

Preparation time: 25 min

Cooking time: 40 min

Servings: 12 Ingredients:

Onion, small, chopped (1 piece)

Cheeseburger macaroni, prepared (1 package)

Salsa, chunky, thick (1 cup)

Cheddar cheese, shredded (1 ½ cups)

Ground beef, lean (1 pound)

Hot water (1 1/3 cups)

195

Milk (1/2 cup)

Flour tortillas, six-inch (6 pieces)

Directions:

Preheat air fryer to 325 degrees fahrenheit.

Cook onion and beef in skillet heated on medium-high until browned. Stir in salsa, hot water, milk, sauce mix, and uncooked pasta. Let mixture boil, then simmer, covered, until pasta is tenderly cooked.

Slice each tortilla in half.

Cover bottom of a baking dish with beef mixture (2 cups), then top with 6 tortilla halves, cheese (3/4 cup), beef mixture (2 cups), and remaining tortilla halves, beef mixture, and finally cheese.

Air-fry for thirty minutes.

Nutrition: calories 265

Fat 30.0 g

Protein 53.0 g

Carbohydrates 18.0 g

206) Baked salsa beef

Preparation time: 15 min

Cooking time: 25 min

Servings: 6

Ingredients:

Salsa, chunky, thick (16 ounces)

Milk (3/4 cup)

Cheddar cheese, shredded (1 cup)

Ground beef, lean (1 pound)

Biscuit mix (2 cups)

Green onion, medium, chopped (1 piece)

Directions:

Preheat air fryer to 375 degrees fahrenheit.

Mist cooking spray onto a square pan. Cook beef until browned; drain before stirring in salsa, then spread in pan. Stir together biscuit mix, cheese, onion, and milk to form a soft dough. Drop 12 tablespoons of dough on top of beef mixture in pan.

Air-fry for twenty-five minutes.

Nutrition: calories 212

Fat 30.0 g

Protein 53.0 g

Carbohydrates 18.0 g

207) Steak and philly cheese biscuit bake

Preparation time: 40 min

Cooking time: 40 min

Servings: 16

Ingredients:

Green bell peppers, medium, sliced thinly into strips (2 pieces)

Steak seasoning (1 tablespoon) Cheese blend, mozzarella & provolone, shredded (2 cups)

Onions, sliced thinly (2 cups)

Biscuits, refrigerated, flaky layers (16 1/3 ounces)

Ground beef, lean (1 pound)

Vegetable oil (1 tablespoon)

Velveeta, original, cubed (8 ounces)

Milk (1 cup) Directions:

Preheat air fryer to 325 degrees fahrenheit.

Mist cooking spray onto a baking dish. Cook beef mixed with steak seasoning until browned. Drain and set aside in a bowl.

Wipe-clean skillet and fill with vegetable oil. Heat on medium-high, stir in bell peppers and onions. Cook until browned before adding to beef bowl.

Melt together cubed cheese, milk, and shredded cheese (1 cup); stir until smooth.

Separate and cut dough to form 6 portions out of each of 8 biscuits. Stir into melted cheese mixture. Add to beef mixture and mix well. Pour into baking dish and top with remaining shredded cheese (1 cup).

Air-fry for thirty-two to thirty-six minutes.

Nutrition: calories 255

Fat 14.0 g

Protein 32.0 g

Carbohydrates 12.0 g

208) Beefy stroganoff casserole

Preparation time: 25 min

Cooking time: 45 min

Servings: 6

Ingredients:

Nutmeg (1/2 teaspoon)
Ground beef, lean (1 pound)
Pepper (1/4 teaspoon)
Garlic cloves, minced (2 pieces)
Sour cream (8 ounces)
Egg noodles, medium, uncooked (8 ounces)
Mushrooms, whole, fresh, small, halved (12 ounces)
Gravy mix, beef/pork (2 ounces)
Water (2 1 2cups)
Parsley, fresh, chopped (1/4 cup)

Directions:

Preheat air fryer to 350 degrees fahrenheit.
Mist cooking spray onto a casserole.

Follow package directions in cooking egg noodles. Drain and keep warm by covering.

Cook beef, garlic, and mushrooms until browned and fully cooked. Drain and set aside. Add to same skillet water, pepper, and gravy mix. Stir and cook until bubbling and thickened. Turn off heat before stirring in nutmeg and sour cream.

Toss cooked noodles with gravy and beef mixture; add to casserole. Cover and airfry for thirty to forty minutes.

Serve sprinkled with parsley.

Nutrition: calories 360

Fat 14.0 g

Protein 32.0 g

Carbohydrates 12.0 g

209) Marinated flank steak

Preparation time: 10 minutes
cooking time: 15 minutes

Servings: 4

Ingredients

¾ lb. Flank steak

1 ½ tbsp. Sake

1 tbsp. Brown miso paste

1 tsp. Honey

2 cloves garlic, pressed

1 tbsp. Olive oil

Directions:

Put all the ingredients in a ziploc bag. Shake to cover the steak well with the seasonings and refrigerate for at least 1 hour. Coat all sides of the steak with cooking spray. Put the steak in the air fryer baking pan. Cook at 400°f for 12 minutes, turning the steak twice during the cooking time, then serve immediately.

Nutrition: calories 255 Fat 14.0 g

Protein 32.0 g Carbohydrates 12.0 g

210) Fried steak

Preparation time: 10 minutes cooking time: 15 minutes

servings: 1

Ingredients

3 cm-thick beef steak   Pepper

and salt to taste

Directions:

Pre-heat the air fryer 400°f for 5 minutes.

Place the beef steak in the baking tray and sprinkle on pepper and salt.

Spritz the steak with cooking spray.

Allow to cook for 3 minutes. Turn the steak over and cook on the other side for 3 more minutes. Serve hot.

Nutrition: calories 255

Fat 14.0 g

Protein 32.0 g

Carbohydrates 12.0 g

211) Homemade meatballs

Preparation time: 10 minutes cooking time: 20 minutes

servings: 4

Ingredients

1 lb. Ground beef

1 tsp. Red thai curry paste

½ lime, rind and juice

1 tsp. Chinese spice

2 tsp. Lemongrass, finely chopped

1 tbsp. Sesame oil

Directions:

Mix all the ingredients in a bowl, combining well. Take 24 equal amounts of the mixture and shape each one into a meatball. Put them in the air fryer cooking basket. Cook at 380°f for 10 minutes. Turn them over and cook for a further 5 minutes on the other side, ensuring they are well-cooked before serving with your favorite dipping sauce. Nutrition: calories 255 Fat 14.0 g

Protein 32.0 g Carbohydrates 12.0 g

212) Crumbed filet mignon

Preparation time: 10 minutes cooking time: 20 minutes

 servings: 4

Ingredients

½ lb. Filet mignon

Sea salt and ground black pepper, to taste

½ tsp. Cayenne pepper

1 tsp. Dried basil

1 tsp. Dried rosemary

1 tsp. Dried thyme

1 tbsp. Sesame oil

1 small-sized egg, well-whisked

½ cup friendly breadcrumbs

Directions:

Cover the filet mignon with the salt, black pepper, cayenne pepper, basil, rosemary, and thyme. Coat with a light brushing of sesame oil.

Put the egg in a shallow plate.

Pour the friendly breadcrumbs in another plate.

Dip the filet mignon into the egg. Roll it into the crumbs.

Transfer the steak to the air fryer and cook for 10 to 13 minutes at 360°f or until it turns golden.

Serve with a salad.

Nutrition: calories 322

Fat 14.0 g

Protein 32.0 g

Carbohydrates 12.0 g

213) Grilled beef ribs

Preparation time: 10 minutes   cooking time: 20 minutes   marinating   time   servings: 4

Ingredients

1 lb. Meaty beef ribs

3 tbsp. Apple cider vinegar

1 cup coriander, finely chopped

1 heaped tbsp. Fresh basil leaves, chopped

2 garlic cloves, finely chopped

1 chipotle powder

1 tsp. Fennel seeds

1 tsp. Hot paprika

Kosher salt and black pepper, to taste

½ cup vegetable oil   Directions:

Wash and dry the ribs.

Coat the ribs with the rest of the ingredients and refrigerate for a minimum of 3 hours.

Separate the ribs from the marinade and put them on an air fryer grill pan.

Cook at 360°f for 8 minutes, or longer as needed.

Pour the remaining marinade over the ribs before serving immediately.

Nutrition: calories 255 Fat 14.0 g

Protein 32.0 g Carbohydrates 12.0 g

214) London broil

Preparation time: 10 minutes   cooking time: 30 minutes   marinating   time   servings: 8

Ingredients

2 lb. London broil

3 large garlic cloves, minced

3 tbsp. Balsamic vinegar

3 tbsp. Whole-grain mustard

2 tbsp. Olive oil

Sea salt and ground black pepper, to taste

½ tsp. Dried hot red pepper flakes

Directions:

Wash and dry the london broil. Score its sides with a knife.

Mix together the rest of the ingredients. Rub this mixture into the broil, coating it well. Allow to marinate for a minimum of 3 hours.

Cook the meat at 400°f for 15 minutes.

Turn it over and cook for an additional 10 - 12 minutes before serving.

Nutrition: calories 255

Fat 14.0 g

Protein 32.0 g

Carbohydrates 12.0 g

215) Smoked beef roast

Preparation time: 10 minutes   cooking time: 45 minutes

 servings: 8

Ingredients

2 lb. Roast beef, at room temperature

2 tbsp. Extra-virgin olive oil

1 tsp. Sea salt flakes

1 tsp. Black pepper, preferably freshly ground

1 tsp. Smoked paprika

Few dashes of liquid smoke

2 jalapeño peppers, thinly sliced

Directions:

Pre-heat the air fryer to 330°f.

With kitchen towels, pat the beef dry.

Massage the extra-virgin olive oil and seasonings into the meat. Cover with liquid smoke.

Place the beef in the air fryer and roast for 30 minutes. Flip the roast over and allow to cook for another 15 minutes.

When cooked through, serve topped with sliced jalapeños.

Nutrition: calories 353

Fat 14.0 g

Protein 32.0 g

Carbohydrates 12.0 g

216) Vegetables & beef cubes

Preparation time: 10 minutes   cooking time: 20 minutes   marinating   time servings: 4

Ingredients

1 lb. Top round steak, cut into cubes

2 tbsp. Olive oil

1 tbsp. Apple cider vinegar

1 tsp. Fine sea salt

½ tsp. Ground black pepper

1 tsp. Shallot powder

¾ tsp. Smoked cayenne pepper

½ tsp. Garlic powder

¼ tsp. Ground cumin

¼ lb. Broccoli, cut into florets

¼ lb. Mushrooms, sliced

1 tsp. Dried basil 1

tsp. Celery seeds

Directions:

Massage the olive oil, vinegar, salt, black pepper, shallot powder, cayenne pepper, garlic powder, and cumin into the cubed steak, ensuring to coat each piece evenly.

Allow to marinate for a minimum of 3 hours.

Put the beef cubes in the air fryer cooking basket and allow to cook at 365°f for 12 minutes.

When the steak is cooked through, place it in a bowl.

Wipe the grease from the cooking basket and pour in the vegetables. Season them with basil and celery seeds.

Cook at 400°f for 5 to 6 minutes. When the vegetables are hot, serve them with the steak.

Nutrition: calories 432

Fat 14.0 g

Protein 32.0 g

Carbohydrates 12.0 g

217) Beef & kale omelet

Preparation time: 10 minutes   cooking time: 20 minutes

 servings: 4

Ingredients

Cooking spray

½ lb. Leftover beef, coarsely chopped

2 garlic cloves, pressed

1 cup kale, torn into pieces and wilted

1 tomato, chopped

¼ tsp. Sugar

4 eggs, beaten

4 tbsp. Heavy cream

½ tsp. Turmeric powder

Salt and ground black pepper to taste

1/8 tsp. Ground allspice

Directions:

Grease four ramekins with cooking spray.

Place equal amounts of each of the ingredients into each ramekin and mix well.

Air-fry at 360°f for 16 minutes, or longer if necessary. Serve immediately.

Nutrition: calories 357

Fat 14.0 g

Protein 32.0 g Carbohydrates 12.0 g

218) Simple beef

Preparation time: 10 minutes   cooking time: 25 minutes

 servings: 1

Ingredients

1 thin beef schnitzel

1 egg, beaten

½ cup friendly breadcrumbs

2 tbsp. Olive oil Pepper and

   salt to taste Directions:

Pre-heat the air fryer to 350°f.

In a shallow dish, combine the breadcrumbs, oil, pepper, and salt.

In a second shallow dish, place the beaten egg.

Dredge the schnitzel in the egg before rolling it in the breadcrumbs.

Put the coated schnitzel in the fryer basket and air fry for 12 minutes.

Meatloaf

Preparation time: 10 minutes cooking time: 30 minutes
 servings: 4

Ingredients

1 lb. Ground beef

1 egg, beaten

1 mushroom, sliced

1 tbsp. Thyme

1 small onion, chopped

3 tbsp. Friendly breadcrumbs

Pepper to taste

Directions:

Pre-heat the air fryer at 400°f. Place all the ingredients into a large bowl and combine entirely. Transfer the meatloaf mixture into the loaf pan and move it to the air fryer basket. Cook for 25 minutes. Slice up before serving.

Nutrition: calories 255 Fat 14.0 g

Protein 32.0 g Carbohydrates 12.0 g

219) Beef burgers

Preparation time: 10

cooking time: 65 servings: 4

Place the diced onion in the fryer and fry until they turn golden brown.

Mix in all the seasoning and cook for 25 minutes at 390°f.

Ingredients

10.5 oz. Beef, minced

1 onion, diced

1 tsp. Garlic, minced or pureed

1 tsp. Tomato, pureed

1 tsp. Mustard

1 tsp. Basil

1 tsp. Mixed herbs

Salt to taste

Pepper to taste

1 oz. Cheddar cheese

4 buns

Salad leaves

Directions:

Drizzle the air fryer with one teaspoon of olive oil and allow it to warm up.

Lay 2 – 3 onion rings and pureed tomato on two of the buns. Place one slice of cheese and the layer of beef on top. Top with salad leaves and any other condiments you desire before closing off the sandwich with the other buns.

Serve with ketchup, cold drink and french fries.

Nutrition: calories 358

Fat 14.0 g

Protein 32.0 g

Carbohydrates 12.0 g

minutes minutes

220) Brussels sprouts & tender beef chuck

Preparation time: 10 minutes   cooking time: 25 minutes   marinating   time

 servings: 4

Ingredients

1 lb. Beef chuck shoulder steak

2 tbsp. Vegetable oil

1 tbsp. Red wine vinegar

1 tsp. Fine sea salt

½ tsp. Ground black pepper

1 tsp. Smoked paprika

1 tsp. Onion powder

½ tsp. Garlic powder

½ lb. Brussels sprouts, cleaned and halved

½ tsp. Fennel seeds

1 tsp. Dried basil 1

tsp. Dried sage

Directions:

Massage the beef with the vegetable oil, wine vinegar, salt, black pepper, paprika, onion powder, and garlic powder, coating it well.

Allow to marinate for a minimum of 3 hours.

Air fry at 390°f for 10 minutes.

Put the prepared brussels sprouts in the fryer along with the fennel seeds, basil, and sage.

Lower the heat to 380°f and cook everything for another 5 minutes.

Pause the machine and give the contents a good stir. Cook for an additional 10 minutes.

Take out the beef and allow the vegetables too cook for a few more minutes if necessary or desired.

Serve everything together with the sauce of your choice.

Nutrition: calories 255 Fat 14.0 g

Protein 32.0 g Carbohydrates 12.0 g

221) Swedish meatballs

Preparation time: 10 cooking time: 25 servings: 8

Ingredients

1 lb. Ground beef

2 friendly bread slices, crumbled

1 small onion, minced

½ tsp. Garlic salt

1 cup tomato sauce

2 cups pasta sauce

1 egg, beaten

2 carrots, shredded Pepper and salt

  to taste Directions:

Pre-heat air fryer to 400°f.

In a bowl, combine the ground beef, egg, carrots, crumbled bread, onion, garlic salt, pepper and salt.

Divide the mixture into equal amounts and shape each one into a small meatball.

Put them in the air fryer basket and cook for 7 minutes.

Transfer the meatballs to an oven-safe dish and top with the tomato sauce.

Set the dish into the air fryer basket and allow to cook at 320°f for 5 more minutes. Serve hot.

Nutrition: calories 255

Fat 14.0 g

Protein 32.0 g

Carbohydrates 12.0 g

222) German schnitzel

Preparation time: 10 minutes   cooking time: 15 minutes

 servings: 4

Ingredients

4 thin beef schnitzel

1 tbsp. Sesame seeds

2 tbsp. Paprika

3 tbsp. Olive oil

minutes minutes

4 tbsp. Flour

2 eggs, beaten

1 cup friendly breadcrumbs

Pepper and salt to taste Directions:

Pre-heat the air fryer at 350°f.

Sprinkle the pepper and salt on the schnitzel.

In a shallow dish, combine the paprika, flour, and salt

In a second shallow dish, mix the breadcrumbs with the sesame seeds.

Place the beaten eggs in a bowl.

Coat the schnitzel in the flour mixture. Dip it into the egg before rolling it in the breadcrumbs.

Put the coated schnitzel in the air fryer basket and allow to cook for 12 minutes before serving hot.

Nutrition: calories 353

Fat 14.0 g

Protein 32.0 g Carbohydrates 12.0 g

223) Steak total

Preparation time: 10 cooking time: 30 servings: 4

Ingredients

2 lb. Rib eye steak

1 tbsp. Olive oil 1

tbsp. Steak rub

Directions:

Set the air fryer to 400°f and allow to warm for 4 minutes.

Massage the olive oil and steak rub into both sides of the steak.

Put the steak in the fryer's basket and cook for 14 minutes. Turn the steak over and cook on the other side for another 7 minutes.

Serve hot.

Nutrition: calories 255 Fat 14.0 g

Protein 32.0 g

Carbohydrates 12.0 g

224) Betty's beef roast

Preparation time: 10 cooking time: 65

servings: 6

Ingredients

2 lb. Beef

1 tbsp. Olive oil

1 tsp. Dried rosemary

1 tsp. Dried thyme

½ tsp. Black pepper

½ tsp. Oregano

½ tsp. Garlic powder

1 tsp. Salt

1 tsp. Onion powder

Directions:

Preheat the air fryer to 330°f.

In a small bowl, mix together all the spices.

minutes

minutes

Coat the beef with a brushing of olive oil.

Massage the spice mixture into the beef.

Transfer the meat to the air fryer and cook for 30 minutes. Turn it over and cook on the other side for another 25 minutes.

Nutrition: calories 255

Fat 14.0 g

Protein 32.0 g

Carbohydrates 12.0 g

225) Beef meatloaf

Preparation time: 10 minutes cooking time: 30 minutes

servings: 4

Ingredients

¾ lb. Ground chuck

¼ lb. Ground pork sausage

1 cup shallots, finely chopped

minutes minutes

2 eggs, well beaten

3 tbsp. Plain milk

1 tbsp. Oyster sauce

1 tsp. Porcini mushrooms

½ tsp. Cumin powder

1 tsp. Garlic paste

1 tbsp. Fresh parsley

Seasoned salt and crushed red pepper flakes to taste 1 cup crushed saltines

Directions:

Mix together all the ingredients in a large bowl, combining everything well.

Transfer to the air fryer baking dish and cook at 360°f for 25 minutes.

Serve hot.

Nutrition: calories 255

Fat 14.0 g

Protein 32.0 g

Carbohydrates 12.0 g

226) Stuffed bell pepper

Preparation time: 10 cooking time: 25 servings: 4

Ingredients

4 bell peppers, cut top of bell pepper

16 oz. Ground beef

2/3 cup cheese, shredded

½ cup rice, cooked

1 tsp. Basil, dried

½ tsp. Chili powder

1 tsp. Black pepper

1 tsp. Garlic salt

2 tsp. Worcestershire sauce

Oz. Tomato sauce

minutes

minutes

2 garlic cloves, minced 1

small onion, chopped

Directions:

Grease a frying pan with cooking spray and fry the onion and garlic over a medium heat.

Stir in the beef, basil, chili powder, black pepper, and garlic salt, combining everything well. Allow to cook until the beef is nicely browned, before taking the pan off the heat.

Add in half of the cheese, the rice, worcestershire sauce, and tomato sauce and stir to combine.

Spoon equal amounts of the beef mixture into the four bell peppers, filling them entirely.

Pre-heat the air fryer at 400°f.

Spritz the air fryer basket with cooking spray.

Put the stuffed bell peppers in the basket and allow to cook for 11 minutes.

Add the remaining cheese on top of each bell pepper with remaining cheese and cook for a further 2 minutes. When the cheese is melted and the bell peppers are piping hot, serve immediately.

Nutrition: calories 255

Fat 14.0 g

Protein 32.0 g Carbohydrates 12.0 g

227) Asian beef burgers

Preparation time: 10 minutes   cooking time: 20 minutes

 servings: 4

Ingredients

¾ lb. Lean ground beef

1 tbsp. Soy sauce

1 tsp. Dijon mustard

Few dashes of liquid smoke

1 tsp. Shallot powder

1 clove garlic, minced

½ tsp. Cumin powder

¼ cup scallions, minced

⅓ tsp. Sea salt flakes

⅓ tsp. Freshly cracked mixed peppercorns

1 tsp. Celery seeds 1 tsp. Parsley flakes

Directions:

Mix together all the ingredients in a bowl using your hands, combining everything well.

minutes

minutes

Take four equal amounts of the mixture and mold each one into a patty.

Use the back of a spoon to create a shallow dip in the center of each patty. This will prevent them from puffing up during the cooking process.

Lightly coat all sides of the patties with cooking spray.

Place each one in the air fryer and cook for roughly 12 minutes at 360°f.

Test with a meat thermometer – the patties are ready once they have reached 160°f. Serve them on top of butter rolls with any sauces and toppings you desire.

Nutrition: calories 255

Fat 14.0 g

Protein 32.0 g

Carbohydrates 12.0 g

228) Burger patties

Preparation time: 10 cooking time: 15 servings: 6

Ingredients

1 lb. Ground beef

6 cheddar cheese slices

Pepper and salt to taste Directions:

Pre-heat the air fryer to 350°f.

Sprinkle the salt and pepper on the ground beef.

Shape six equal portions of the ground beef into patties and put each one in the air fryer basket.

Air fry the patties for 10 minutes.

Top the patties with the cheese slices and air fry for one more minute.

Serve the patties on top of dinner rolls.

Nutrition: calories 255 Fat 14.0 g

Protein 32.0 g Carbohydrates 12.0 g

229) Beef rolls

Preparation time: 10 minutes   cooking time: 30 minutes

 servings: 2

Ingredients

2 lb. Beef flank steak

3 tsp. Pesto

1 tsp. Black pepper

6 slices of provolone cheese

3 oz. Roasted red bell peppers

¾ cup baby spinach

1 tsp. Sea salt

Directions:

Spoon equal amounts of the pesto onto each flank steak and spread it across evenly.

Place the cheese, roasted red peppers and spinach on top of the meat, about three-quarters of the way down.

Roll the steak up, holding it in place with toothpicks. Sprinkle on the sea salt and pepper.

Place inside the air fryer and cook for 14 minutes at 400°f, turning halfway through the cooking time.

Allow the beef to rest for 10 minutes before slicing up and serving.

Nutrition: calories 255

Fat 14.0 g

Protein 32.0 g

Carbohydrates 12.0 g

230) Air fried steak

Preparation time: 5 minutes

Cooking time: 15 minutes

Servings: 4 Ingredients

1.5 pounds rib eye steak

Salt and pepper to taste

A dash of rosemary

½ tablespoon garlic powder

minutes

minutes

3 tablespoons olive oil

Directions:

Place all ingredients in a ziploc bag and marinate in the fridge for at least 2 hours.

Preheat the air fryer at 4000f for 5 minutes.

Place the steak in the air fryer and cook for 15 minutes at 4000f.

Serve hot and enjoy.

Nutrition: calories 255

Fat 14.0 g

Protein 32.0 g

Carbohydrates 12.0 g

231) Air fried beef schnitzel

Preparation time: 5 minutes

Cooking time: 15 minutes

Servings: 1

Ingredients

2 tablespoons vegetable oil

½ cup almond flour

4 ounces shoulder steak or topside cut, thinly sliced

1 large egg, beaten 1 slice

of lemon, to serve

Directions:

Preheat the air fryer at 3500f for 5 minutes.

Mix the oil and almond flour together.

Dip the schnitzel into the egg and dredge in the almond flour mixture.

Press the almond flour so that it sticks on to the beef.

Place in the air fryer and cook for 15 minutes at 3500f.

Serve with a slice of lemon. Enjoy!

Nutrition: calories 952

Fat 14.0 g

Protein 32.0 g

Carbohydrates 12.0 g

232) Air fryer beef casserole

Preparation time: 5 minutes

Cooking time: 30 minutes

Servings: 8

Ingredients

1-pound ground beef (85% lean, 15% fat)

1 medium onion, chopped

3 cloves of garlic, minced

3 tablespoons olive oil

1 green bell pepper, seeded and chopped

Salt and pepper to taste

12 large eggs, beaten

Directions:

Preheat the air fryer at 3250f for 5 minutes.

In a baking dish that will fit in the air fryer, mix the ground beef, onion, garlic, olive oil, and bell pepper. Season with salt and pepper to taste.

Pour in the beaten eggs and give a good stir.

Place the dish with the beef and egg mixture in the air fryer.

Bake for 30 minutes at 3250f.

Serve and enjoy!

Nutrition: calories: 317

Carbohydrates: 3 g

Protein: 25.1 g

Fat: 22.1 g

Sugar: 1.3 g

Sodium: 159 mg

Fiber: 0.4 g

233) Air fried steak with oregano

Preparation time: 5 minutes

Cooking time: 15 minutes

Servings: 4

Ingredients

1-pound beef steak, bones removed

3 tablespoons heart-healthy oil

Salt and pepper to taste

A dash of oregano

Directions:

Place all ingredients in a ziploc bag and marinate in the fridge for at least 2 hours.

Preheat the air fryer at 4000f for 5 minutes.

Place the steak in the air fryer and cook for 15 minutes at 4000f. Serve and enjoy!

Nutrition: calories: 443

Carbohydrates: 3 g

Protein: 25.1 g

Fat: 22.1 g

Sugar: 1.3 g

Sodium: 159 mg

Fiber: 0.4 g

234) Beef pot pie

Preparation time: 10 minutes

Cooking time: 30 minutes

Servings: 6

Ingredients

1-pound ground beef

1 green bell pepper, julienned

1 red bell pepper, julienned

1 yellow bell pepper, julienned

1 medium onion, chopped

2 cloves of garlic, minced

4 tablespoons heart-healthy oil

1 tablespoon butter

Salt and pepper to taste

1 cup almond flour 2

large eggs, beaten

Directions:

Preheat the air fryer at 3500f for 5 minutes.

In a baking dish that will fit in the air fryer, combine the first 9 ingredients. Mix well then set aside.

In a mixing bowl, mix the almond flour and eggs to create a dough.

Press the dough over the beef mixture.

Place in the air fryer and cook for 30 minutes at 3500f.

Serve and enjoy!

Nutrition: calories: 317

Carbohydrates: 3 g

Protein: 25.1 g

Fat: 22.1 g

Sugar: 1.3 g

Sodium: 159 mg

Fiber: 0.4 g

235) Perfect air fried roast beef

Preparation time: 5 minutes

Cooking time: 1 hour

Serve and enjoy!

Nutrition: calories: 387

Carbohydrates: 3 g

Servings: 8

Ingredients

2 pounds topside of beef

2 medium onions, chopped

2 celery stalks, sliced

1 garlic clove, minced

A bunch of fresh herbs of your choice

Salt and pepper to taste

3 tablespoons olive oil

1 tablespoon butter

Directions:

Preheat the air fryer at 3500f for 5 minutes.

Place all the ingredients in a baking dish that will fit in the air fryer and stir.

Place the dish in the air fryer and bake for 1 hour at 3500f.

1 medium onion, chopped

3 celery stalks, sliced

1 teaspoon thyme

Protein: 25.1 g

Fat: 22.1 g

Sugar: 1.3 g

Sodium: 159 mg

Fiber: 0.4 g

236) Air fried braised beef roast

Preparation time: 5 minutes

Cooking time: 2 hours

Servings: 4

Ingredients

1-pound beef chuck roast

2 tablespoons olive oil

1 tablespoon butter

1 tablespoon worcestershire sauce

2 cloves of garlic, minced

1 teaspoon rosemary

3 cups water

Directions:

Preheat the air fryer at 3500f for 5 minutes.

Place all ingredients in a deep baking dish that will fit in the air fryer.

Bake for 2 hours at 3500f.

Braise the meat with its sauce every 30 minutes until cooked.

Serve and enjoy!

Nutrition: calories: 317

Carbohydrates: 3 g

Protein: 25.1 g

Fat: 22.1 g Sugar: 1.3 g

Sodium: 159 mg

Fiber: 0.4 g

237) Texas beef brisket

Preparation time: 5 minutes

Cooking time: 1 hour and 30 minutes

Servings: 8

Ingredients

2 tablespoons chili powder

1 tablespoon garlic powder

1 tablespoon onion powder

2 teaspoons dry mustard

1 bay leaf

4 tablespoons olive oil

2 pounds beef brisket, trimmed

Salt and pepper to taste

1 ½ cup beef stock

Directions:

Preheat the air fryer at 4000f for 5 minutes.

Place all ingredients in a deep baking dish that will fit in the air fryer.

Bake for 1 hour and 30 minutes at 4000f.

Stir the beef after every 30 minutes to soak in the sauce.

Serve and enjoy!

Nutrition information:

Nutrition: calories: 317

Carbohydrates: 3 g

Protein: 25.1 g

Fat: 22.1 g

Sugar: 1.3 g

Sodium: 159 mg

Fiber: 0.4 g

238) Air fried grilled steak

Preparation time: 5 minutes

Cooking time: 45 minutes

Servings: 2

Ingredients

8 ounces top sirloin steak

2 tablespoons olive oil

½ tablespoon garlic powder

Salt and pepper to taste   2 tablespoons butter, melted

Directions:

Preheat the air fryer at 3500f for 5 minutes.

Season the sirloin steaks with olive oil, garlic powder, salt and pepper.

Place the beef in the air fryer basket.

Cook for 45 minutes at 3500f.

Once cooked, serve with butter. Enjoy!

Nutrition: calories: 317

Carbohydrates: 3 g

Protein: 25.1 g

Fat: 22.1 g

Sugar: 1.3 g

Sodium: 159 mg

Fiber: 0.4 g

239) Barbecued beef brisket

Preparation time: 5 minutes

Cooking time: 2 hours

Servings: 12

Ingredients

1 ½ tablespoons paprika

2 teaspoons dry mustard

2 teaspoons ground black pepper

2 teaspoons salt

1 teaspoon onion powder

1 teaspoon garlic powder

1 teaspoon ground cumin

¼ teaspoon cayenne pepper

3 pounds brisket roast

5 tablespoons olive oil

Directions:

Place all ingredients in a ziploc bag and marinate in the fridge for at least 2 hours.

Preheat the air fryer at 3500f for 5 minutes.

Place the meat in a baking dish that will fit in the air fryer.

Place in the air fryer and cook for 2 hours at 3500f.

Serve and enjoy!

Nutrition: calories: 395

Carbohydrates: 3 g

Protein: 25.1 g

Fat: 22.1 g

Sugar: 1.3 g

Sodium: 159 mg

Fiber: 0.4 g

240) Oven-braised corned beef

Preparation time: 5 minutes

Cooking time: 50 minutes

Servings: 12

Ingredients

4 cups water

3 pounds corned beef brisket, cut into chunks

2 tablespoons dijon mustard

1 medium onion, chopped

Salt and pepper to taste

Directions:

Preheat the air fryer at 4000f for 5 minutes.

Place all ingredients in a baking dish that will fit in the air fryer.

Cook for 50 minutes at 4000f.

Serve and enjoy!

Nutrition: calories: 317

Carbohydrates: 3 g

Protein: 25.1 g

Fat: 22.1 g

Sugar: 1.3 g

Sodium: 159 mg

Fiber: 0.4 g

241) Herb-rubbed top round roast

Preparation time: 5 minutes

Cooking time: 1 hour

Servings: 16

Ingredients

4 pounds beef top round roast

3 tablespoons olive oil

4 teaspoons dried oregano

4 teaspoons dried thyme

2 teaspoons dried rosemary

Salt and pepper to taste

1 teaspoon dry mustard

Directions:

Preheat the air fryer at 3250f for 5 minutes.

Place all ingredients in a baking dish that will fit in the air fryer.

Place the dish in the air fryer and cook for 1 hour at 3250f.

Serve and enjoy!

Nutrition: calories: 317

Carbohydrates: 3 g

Protein: 25.1 g

Fat: 22.1 g

Sugar: 1.3 g

Sodium: 159 mg

Fiber: 0.4 g

242) Air fried roast beef

Preparation time: 5 minutes

Cooking time: 2 hours

Servings: 10

Ingredients

3 pounds bone-in beef roast

1 large onion, quartered

1 tablespoon fresh thyme

1 tablespoon fresh rosemary

3 cups beef broth

2 tablespoons worcestershire sauce

Salt and pepper to taste

4 tablespoons olive oil

Directions:

Preheat the air fryer at 3250f for 5 minutes.

Place all ingredients in a baking dish that will fit in the air fryer.

Place the dish in the air fryer and cook for 2 hours at 3250f.

Serve and enjoy!

Nutrition: calories: 412

Carbohydrates: 3 g

Protein: 25.1 g

Fat: 22.1 g

Sugar: 1.3 g

Sodium: 159 mg

Fiber: 0.4 g

243) Rosemary pepper beef rib roast

Preparation time: 5 minutes

Cooking time: 2 hours

Servings: 7

Ingredients

3 tablespoons vegetable oil

7 ribs, beef rib roast

3 tablespoons unsalted butter

1 medium shallot, chopped

2 cloves of garlic, minced

2 cups water

3 ounces dried porcini mushrooms

4 sprigs of thyme Salt and pepper to taste

Directions:

Preheat the air fryer at 3250f for 5 minutes.

Place all ingredients in a baking dish that will fit in the air fryer.

Place the dish in the air fryer and cook for 2 hours at 3250f.

Serve and enjoy!

Nutrition: calories: 317

Carbohydrates: 3 g

Protein: 25.1 g

Fat: 22.1 g

Sugar: 1.3 g

Sodium: 159 mg

Fiber: 0.4 g

244) Peppered roast beef with shallots

Preparation time: 5 minutes

Cooking time: 1 hour and 30 minutes

Servings: 12

Ingredients

3 tablespoons mixed peppercorns

3-pound boneless rib roast

4 tablespoons olive oil

Salt to taste

4 medium shallots, chopped

2 tablespoons whole grain mustard

¼ cup flat-leaf parsley, chopped

Directions:

Preheat the air fryer at 3250f for 5 minutes.

Place all ingredients in a baking dish that will fit in the air fryer.

Place the dish in the air fryer and cook for 1 hour and 30 minutes at 3250f.

Serve and enjoy!

Nutrition: calories: 317

Carbohydrates: 3 g

Protein: 25.1 g

Fat: 22.1 g

Sugar: 1.3 g

Sodium: 159 mg

Fiber: 0.4 g

245) Bullet-proof beef roast

Preparation time: 2 hours

Cooking time: 2 hours

Servings: 12

Ingredients

4 tablespoons olive oil

Salt and pepper to taste

1 cup organic beef broth 3

pounds beef round roast

Directions:

Place all the ingredients in a ziploc bag and marinate in the fridge for 2 hours.

Preheat the air fryer at 4000f for 5 minutes.

Transfer all ingredients in a baking dish that will fit in the air fryer.

Place in the air fryer and cook for 2 hours at 4000f.

Serve and enjoy!

Nutrition: calories: 317

Carbohydrates: 3 g

Protein: 25.1 g

Fat: 22.1 g

Sugar: 1.3 g

Sodium: 159 mg

Fiber: 0.4 g

Snacks

246) Pork bites

Preparation time: 10 minutes

Cooking time: 15 minutes

Servings: 4

Ingredients:

2 teaspoons garlic powder

2 eggs

Salt and black pepper to taste

¾ cup panko breadcrumbs

¾ cup coconut, shredded

A drizzle of olive oil   1-pound

ground pork

Directions:

In a bowl, mix coconut with panko and stir well.

In another bowl, mix the pork, salt, pepper, eggs, and garlic powder, and then shape medium meatballs out of this mix.

Dredge the meatballs in the coconut mix, place them in your air fryer's basket, introduce in the air fryer, and cook at 350 degrees f for 15 minutes.

Serve and enjoy!

Nutrition:

calories 192

Fat 4 Fiber 2

carbs 14

Protein 6

247) Banana chips

Preparation time: 5 minutes

Cooking time: 5 minutes

Servings: 8

Ingredients:

¼ cup peanut butter, soft

1 banana, peeled and sliced into 16 pieces

1 tablespoon vegetable oil

Directions:

Put the banana slices in your air fryer's basket and drizzle the oil over them.

Cook at 360 degrees f for 5 minutes.

Transfer to bowls and serve them dipped in peanut butter.

Nutrition values: calories 100, fat 4, fiber 1, carbs 10, protein 4

248) Lemony apple bites

Preparation time: 5 minutes

Cooking time: 5 minutes

Servings: 4

Ingredients:

3 big apples, cored, peeled and cubed

2 teaspoons lemon juice

½ cup caramel sauce

Directions:

In your air fryer, mix all the ingredients; toss well.

Cook at 340 degrees f for 5 minutes.

Divide into cups and serve as a snack.

Nutrition:

calories 190

Fat 4 Fiber 2

carbs 14

Protein 6

249) Zucchini balls

Preparation time: 10 minutes

Cooking time: 12 minutes

Servings: 8

Ingredients:

Cooking spray

½ cup dill, chopped

1 egg

½ cup white flour

Salt and black pepper to taste

2 garlic cloves, minced

3 zucchinis, grated

Directions:

In a bowl, mix all the ingredients and stir.

Shape the mix into medium balls and place them into your air fryer's basket.

Cook at 375 degrees f for 12 minutes, flipping them halfway.

Serve them as a snack right away.

Nutrition:

calories 120

Fat 4 Fiber 2

carbs 14

Protein 6

250) Basil and cilantro crackers

Preparation time: 10 minutes

Cooking time: 16 minutes

Servings: 6

Ingredients:

½ teaspoon baking powder

Salt and black pepper to taste

1¼ cups flour

1 garlic clove, minced

2 tablespoons basil, minced

2 tablespoons cilantro, minced

4 tablespoons butter, melted

Directions:

Add all the ingredients to a bowl and stir until you obtain a dough.

Spread this on a lined baking sheet that fits your air fryer.

Place the baking sheet in the fryer at 325 degrees f and cook for 16 minutes.

Cool down, cut, and serve.

Nutrition:

calories 171

Keto Air Fryer Cookbook For Beginners

Fat 4 Fiber 2

carbs 14

Protein 6

251) Balsamic zucchini slices

Preparation time: 5 minutes

Cooking time: 50 minutes

Servings: 6

Ingredients:

3 zucchinis, thinly sliced

Salt and black pepper to taste

2 tablespoons avocado oil   2 tablespoons balsamic vinegar

Directions:

Add all the ingredients to a bowl and mix.

Put the zucchini mixture in your air fryer's basket and cook at 220 degrees f for 50 minutes.

Serve as a snack and enjoy!

Nutrition:

calories 40

Fat 4 Fiber

2 carbs 14

Protein 6

252) Turmeric carrot chips

Preparation time: 5 minutes

Cooking time: 25 minutes

Servings: 4

Ingredients:

4 carrots, thinly sliced

Salt and black pepper to taste

½ teaspoon turmeric powder

½ teaspoon chat masala

1 teaspoon olive oil

Directions:

Place all ingredients in a bowl and toss well.

Put the mixture in your air fryer's basket and cook at 370 degrees f for 25 minutes, shaking the fryer from time to time.

Serve as a snack.

Nutrition: calories

161 Fat 4 Fiber 2

carbs 14 Protein 6

253) Chives radish snack

Preparation time: 5 minutes

Cooking time: 10 minutes

Servings: 4

Ingredients:

16 radishes, sliced

A drizzle of olive oil

Salt and black pepper to taste

1 tablespoon chives, chopped

Directions:

In a bowl, mix the radishes, salt, pepper, and oil; toss well.

Place the radishes in your air fryer's basket and cook at 350 degrees f for 10 minutes.

Divide into bowls and serve with chives sprinkled on top.

Nutrition:

calories 192

Fat 4 Fiber 2

carbs 14

Protein 6

254) Lentils snack

Preparation time: 5 minutes

Cooking time: 12 minutes

Servings: 4

Ingredients:

15 ounces canned lentils, drained

½ teaspoon cumin, ground

1 tablespoon olive oil

1 teaspoon sweet paprika   Salt and black pepper to taste

Directions:

Place all ingredients in a bowl and mix well.

Transfer the mixture to your air fryer and cook at 400 degrees f for 12 minutes.

Divide into bowls and serve as a snack or a side, or appetizer!

Nutrition: calories 151 Fat

4 Fiber 2 carbs 14

Protein 6

255) Air fried corn

Preparation time: 5 minutes

Cooking time: 10 minutes

Servings: 4

Ingredients:

2 tablespoons corn kernels

2½ tablespoons butter

Directions:

In a pan that fits your air fryer, mix the corn with the butter.

Place the pan in the fryer and cook at 400 degrees f for 10 minutes.

Serve as a snack and enjoy!

Nutrition:

calories 192

Fat 4 Fiber 2

carbs 14

Protein 6

256) Salmon tarts

Preparation time: 20 min

Cooking time: 10 minutes

Servings: 15

Ingredients

15 mini tart cases

4 eggs, lightly beaten

½ cup heavy cream

Salt and black pepper

3 oz smoked salmon

6 oz cream cheese, divided into 15 pieces

6 fresh dill

Directions

Mix together eggs and cream in a pourable measuring container. Arrange the tarts into the air fryer. Pour in mixture into the tarts, about halfway up the side and top with a piece of salmon and a piece of cheese. Cook for 10 minutes at 340 f, regularly check to avoid overcooking. Sprinkle dill and serve chilled.

Nutrition: calories 415 Fat 4 Fiber 2

carbs 14 Protein 6

257) Parmesan crusted pickles

Preparation time: 35 min

Cooking time: 25 minutes

Servings: 4

Ingredients

3 cups dill pickles, sliced, drained

2 eggs

2 tsp water

1 cup grated parmesan cheese

1 ½ cups breadcrumbs, smooth

Black pepper to taste

Cooking spray

Directions

Add the breadcrumbs and black pepper to a bowl and mix well; set aside. In another bowl, crack the eggs and beat with the water. Set aside. Add the cheese to a separate bowl; set aside. Preheat the air fryer to 400 f.

Pull out the fryer basket and spray it lightly with cooking spray. Dredge the pickle slices it in the egg mixture, then in breadcrumbs and then in cheese. Place them in the fryer without overlapping.

Slide the fryer basket back in and cook for 4 minutes. Turn them and cook for further for 5 minutes, until crispy. Serve with a cheese dip.

Nutrition:

calories 335

Fat 4 Fiber 2

carbs 14

Protein 6

258) Breaded mushrooms

Preparation time: 55 min

Cooking time: 25 minutes

Servings: 4

Ingredients

1 lb. Small button mushrooms, cleaned

2 cups breadcrumbs

2 eggs, beaten

Salt and pepper to taste

2 cups parmigiano reggiano cheese, grated

Directions

Preheat the air fryer to 360 f. Pour the breadcrumbs in a bowl, add salt and pepper and mix well. Pour the cheese in a separate bowl and set aside. Dip each mushroom in the eggs, then in the crumbs, and then in the cheese.

Slide out the fryer basket and add 6 to 10 mushrooms. Cook them for 20 minutes, in batches, if needed. Serve with cheese dip.

Nutrition:

calories 192

Fat 4 Fiber 2

carbs 14

Protein 6

259) Cheesy sticks with sweet thai sauce

Preparation time: 2 hrs. 20 min

Cooking time: 25 minutes

Servings: 4

Ingredients

12 mozzarella string cheese

2 cups breadcrumbs

3 eggs

1 cup sweet thai sauce

4 tbsp skimmed milk

Directions

Pour the crumbs in a medium bowl. Crack the eggs into another bowl and beat with the milk. One after the other, dip each cheese sticks in the egg mixture, in the crumbs, then egg mixture again and then in the crumbs again.

Place the coated cheese sticks on a cookie sheet and freeze for 1 to 2 hours. Preheat the air fryer to 380 f. Arrange the sticks in the fryer without overcrowding. Cook for 5 minutes, flipping them halfway through cooking

to brown evenly. Cook in batches. Serve Stretch the bacon strips to elongate and with a sweet thai sauce. use a knife to cut in half to make 24 Nutrition: pieces. Wrap each bacon piece around a calories 158 slice of avocado from one end to the

other end. Tuck the end of bacon into

Fat 4

the wrap. Arrange on a flat surface and

Fiber 2

carbs 14

Protein 6

260) Bacon wrapped avocados

Preparation time: 40 min

Cooking time: 25 minutes   calories 192

Servings: 6

Ingredients

12 thick strips bacon   carbs 14
3 large avocados, sliced

⅓ tsp salt

⅓ tsp chili powder

⅓ tsp cumin powder

Directions

season with salt, chili and cumin on both sides.

Arrange 4 to 8 wrapped pieces in the fryer and cook at 350 f for 8 minutes, or until the bacon is browned and crunchy, flipping halfway through to cook evenly.

Remove onto a wire rack and repeat the process for the remaining avocado pieces.

Nutrition:

Fat 4

Fiber 2

Protein 6

261) Hot chicken wingettes

Preparation time: 45 min

Cooking time: 30 minutes

Servings: 3

Ingredients

15 chicken wingettes

Salt and pepper to taste

⅓ cup hot sauce

⅓ cup butter

½ tbsp vinegar

Directions

Preheat the air fryer to 360 f. Season the wingettes with pepper and salt. Add them to the air fryer and cook for 35 minutes. Toss every 5 minutes. Once ready, remove them into a bowl. Over low heat, melt the butter in a saucepan. Add the vinegar and hot sauce. Stir and cook for a minute.

Turn the heat off. Pour the sauce over the chicken. Toss to coat well. Transfer the chicken to a serving platter. Serve with a side of celery strips and blue cheese dressing.

Nutrition:

calories

563 Fat 4

Fiber 2

carbs 14

Protein 6

262) Bacon & chicken wrapped jalapenos

Preparation time: 40 min

Cooking time: 30 minutes

Servings: 4

Ingredients

Jalapeno peppers, halved lengthwise and seeded

4 chicken breasts, butterflied and halved

6 oz cream cheese

6 oz cheddar cheese

16 slices bacon

1 cup breadcrumbs

Salt and pepper to taste

2 eggs

Cooking spray

Directions

Season the chicken with pepper and salt on both sides. In a bowl, add cream cheese, cheddar, a pinch of pepper and salt. Mix well. Take each jalapeno and spoon in the cheese mixture to the brim. On a working board, flatten each piece of chicken and lay 2 bacon slices each on them. Place a stuffed jalapeno on each laid out chicken and bacon set and wrap the jalapenos in them.

Preheat the air fryer to 350 f. Add the eggs to a bowl and pour the breadcrumbs in another bowl. Also, set a flat plate aside. Take each wrapped jalapeno and dip it into the eggs and then in the breadcrumbs. Place them on the flat plate. Lightly grease the fryer basket with cooking spray. Arrange 4-5 breaded jalapenos in the basket and cook for 7 minutes.

Prepare a paper towel lined plate; set aside. Once the timer beeps, open the fryer, turn the jalapenos, and cook further for 4 minutes. Once ready, remove them onto the paper towel lined plate. Repeat the cooking process for the remaining jalapenos. Serve with a sweet dip for an enhanced taste.

Nutrition:

calories

192 Fat 4

Fiber 2

carbs 14

Protein 6

263) Mouth-watering salami sticks

Preparation time: 2 hrs. 10 min

Cooking time: 20 minutes

Servings: 3

Ingredients

1 lb. Ground beef

3 tbsp sugar

A pinch garlic powders

A pinch chili powders

Salt to taste

1 tsp liquid smoke

Directions

Place the meat, sugar, garlic powder, chili powder, salt and liquid smoke in a bowl. Mix with a spoon. Mold out 4 sticks with your hands, place them on a plate, and refrigerate for 2 hours. Cook at 350 f. For 10 minutes, flipping once halfway through.

Nutrition:

calories 428

Carbs 12g

Fat 16g

Protein 42g

Nutrition:

calories 35

Carbs 12g

Fat 16g

Protein 42g

264) Carrot crisps

Preparation time: 20 min

Cooking time: 20 minutes

Servings: 2

Ingredients

3 large carrots, washed and peeled

Salt to taste

Cooking spray

Directions

Using a mandolin slicer, slice the carrots very thinly height wise. Put the carrot strips in a bowl and season with salt to taste. Grease the fryer basket lightly with cooking spray and add the carrot strips. Cook at 350 f for 10 minutes, stirring once halfway through.

265) Calamari with olives

Preparation time: 25 min

Cooking time: 30 minutes

Servings: 3

Ingredients

½ lb. Calamari rings

½ piece coriander, chopped

2 strips chili pepper, chopped

1 tbsp olive oil

1 cup pimiento-stuffed green olives, sliced

Salt and black pepper to taste

Directions

In a bowl, add rings, chili pepper, salt, black pepper, oil, and coriander. Mix and let marinate for 10 minutes. Pour the calamari into an oven-safe bowl, that fits into the fryer basket.

Slide the fryer basket out, place the bowl in it, and slide the basket back in. Cook for 15 minutes stirring every 5 minutes using a spoon, at 400 f. After 15 minutes and add in the olives.

Stir, close and continue to cook for 3 minutes. Once ready, transfer to a serving platter. Serve warm with a side of bread slices and mayonnaise.

Nutrition:

calories 128

Carbs 12g

Fat 16g

Protein 42g

266) Sweet mixed nuts

Preparation time: 25 min

Cooking time: 30 minutes

Servings: 5

Ingredients

½ cup pecans

½ cup walnuts

½ cup almonds

A pinch cayenne peppers

2 tbsp sugar

2 tbsp egg whites

2 tsp cinnamon

Cooking spray

Directions

Add the pepper, sugar, and cinnamon to a bowl and mix well; set aside. In another bowl, mix in the pecans, walnuts, almonds, and egg whites. Add the spice mixture to the nuts and give it a good mix. Lightly grease the fryer basket with cooking spray.

Pour in the nuts and cook them for 10 minutes. Stir the nuts using a wooden vessel and cook for further for 10 minutes. Pour the nuts in the bowl. Let cool before crunching on them.

Nutrition:

calories 147

Carbs 12g

Fat 16g

Protein 42g

267) Cheesy onion rings

Preparation time: 20 min

Cooking time: 25 minutes

Servings: 3

Ingredients

1 onion, peeled and sliced into 1-inch rings

¾ cup parmesan cheese

2 medium eggs, beaten

1 tsp garlic powder

A pinch of salt

1 cup flour

1 tsp paprika powder

Directions

Add the eggs to a bowl; set aside in another bowl, add cheese, garlic powder, salt, flour, and paprika. Mix with a spoon. Dip each onion ring in egg, then in the cheese mixture, in the egg again and finally in the cheese mixture.

Add the rings to the basket and cook them for 8 minutes at 350 f. Remove onto a serving platter and serve with a cheese or tomatoes dip.

Nutrition:

calories 205

Carbs 12g

Fat 16g

Protein 42g

268) Cheesy sausage balls

Preparation time: 50 min

Cooking time: 25 minutes

Servings: 8

Ingredients

1 ½ lb. Ground sausages

2 ¼ cups cheddar cheese, shredded

1 ½ cup flour

¾ tsp baking soda

4 eggs

¾ cup sour cream

1 tsp dried oregano

1 tsp smoked paprika

2 tsp garlic powder

½ cup liquid coconut oil

Directions

In a pan over medium heat, add the sausages and brown for 3-4 minutes. Drain the excess fat and set aside. In a bowl, sift in baking soda, and flour. Set aside. In another bowl, add eggs, sour cream, oregano, paprika, coconut oil, and garlic powder. Whisk to combine well. Combine the egg and flour mixtures using a spatula.

Add the cheese and sausages. Fold in and let it sit for 5 minutes to thicken. Rub your hands with coconut oil and mold out bite-size balls out of the batter. Place them on a tray and refrigerate for 15 minutes. Then, add them in the air fryer, without overcrowding. Cook for 10 minutes per round, at 400 f, in batches if needed.

Nutrition:

calories 457

Carbs 12g

Fat 16g

Protein 42g

269) Crusted coconut shrimp

Preparation time: 30 min

Cooking time: 25 minutes

Servings: 5

Ingredients

1 lb. Jumbo shrimp, peeled and deveined

¾ cup shredded coconut

1 tbsp maple syrup

½ cup breadcrumbs

⅓ cup cornstarch

½ cup milk

Directions

Pour the cornstarch in a zipper bag, add shrimp, zip the bag up and shake vigorously to coat with the cornstarch. Mix the syrup and milk in a bowl and set aside. In a separate bowl, mix the breadcrumbs and shredded coconut. Open the zipper bag and remove each shrimp while shaking off excess starch.

Dip each shrimp in the milk mixture and then in the crumbs mixture while pressing loosely to trap enough crumbs and coconut. Place the coated shrimp in the fryer without overcrowding.

Cook 12 minutes at 350 f, flipping once halfway through. Cook until golden brown. Serve with a coconut-based dip.

Nutrition:

calories 428

Carbs 12g

Fat 16g

Protein 42g

270) French fries in instant pot air fryer

Preparation time: 5 minutes

cooking: 12 minutes

Servings: 4

Ingredients:

2 pounds (6 nos.) Parsnips

¼ cup olive oil

¼ cup of water

¼ cup almond flour

1 teaspoon salt Olive

oil cooking spray

Directions:

Wash, peel the parsnips and pat dry before you chop them into ½ inch sizes In a large bowl to mix the almond flour, water, salt, and olive oil. Combine it well until there are no lumps at all.

Add the parsnips to this mix and stir it well until everything gets a proper coating.

Place the coated parsnips in the air fryer basket and put the basket in the inner pot of the instant pot air fryer.

Close the crisp cover.

Now in the air fry mode and set the temperature at 390° f and keep the timer for 12 minutes.

Press start to begin the frying.

It is a good habit if you can open the crisp lid and shake the basket for even cooking.

Spritz some cooking spray while shaking the basket, which can help to improve the crispness.

Keep cooking 2 more minutes if you don't find it crispy enough.

Serve it hot.

Nutrition:

calories 428

Carbs 12g

Fat 16g

Protein 42g

271) Air fryer paleo cauliflower tater tots

Preparation time: 30 minutes

cooking: 15 minutes

Servings: 24 tots

Ingredients: 2-pound (1

nos.) Cauliflower head, large

1 teaspoon parsley, dried

1 teaspoon onion powder

1 teaspoon garlic powder

¼ cup coconut flour

2 eggs, large

1 teaspoon salt

1 teaspoon ground black pepper

Coconut oil spray

Water as required

Directions:

Wash and separate cauliflower into florets.

Pat dry.

Microwave the florets in 2 tablespoons water in an oven-safe bowl.

Cover the bowl and microwave it for around 3-5 minutes until the florets become tender.

Once it becomes tender, transfer the florets in the blender or a chopper and blitz until it turns like rice grain.

In a medium bowl, add the florets mix, stir in the eggs, garlic powder, coconut flour, onion powder, parsley, salt, and pepper. Combine it thoroughly. Now make as many tater tots as possible with the mix.

Place the tots in the refrigerator for at least 30 minutes.

After 30 minutes, remove it from the refrigerator.

Spritz some coconut oil in the air fryer basket and place the tots in the basket.

Spray some coconut oil on the tots.

Place the air fryer basket in the inner pot of the instant pot air fryer.

Close the crisp lid.

In the air fry mode, set the temperature to 400°f and timer to 12 minutes.

Press start to begin the cooking.

Halfway through the cooking, open the crisp cover and shake the basket, and spray some cooking oil for even cooking.

Close the crisp cover, so that the instant pot will continue with the remaining cooking process.

Serve it hot with your choice of sauce.

Nutrition:

calories 16

Carbs 12g

Fat 16g

Protein 42g

272) Air fried asparagus

Preparation time: 5 minutes

cooking: 10 minutes

Servings: 4

Ingredients:

1-pound (½ bunch) asparagus

1 teaspoon ground black pepper

½ teaspoon himalayan salt

1 olive oil spray Directions:

Wash asparagus in running water, pat dry, and trim the bottom. Put the asparagus in the air fryer basket and sprinkle the salt and pepper on it.

Place the air fryer basket in the inner pot of the instant pot air fryer.

Close the crisp cover. In the air fry mode, set the temperature at 400°f and the timer to 10 minutes.

Press the start to begin the cooking. Halfway through the cooking, open the crisp cover, and shake the basket for even cooking.

Close the crisp cover after shaking, so that the appliance can resume the cooking with the same setting.

Once the timer goes off, serve the asparagus hot with the choice of sauces.

Nutrition:

calories 25

Carbs 12g

Fat 16g

Protein 42g

273) Air fried salmon cakes

Preparation time: 10 minutes

Cooking: 25 minutes

Servings: 2

Ingredients:

2 cans (7.5 ounces) salmon, unsalted, with bones and skin 2 lemon wedges

1 egg, large

¼ teaspoon ground black pepper

2 teaspoons mustard, dijon

2 tablespoons of canola mayonnaise

2 tablespoons dill, freshly chopped

½ cup panko breadcrumbs, whole-wheat Vegetable

cooking spray

Directions:

Place the salmon on a flat surface and remove skin and large bone, if any.

Put it in a medium bowl and add dill, panko, mayonnaise, pepper, mustard, and combine gently.   Shape this mixture in cake sizes of 3inch diameter.

Spray some cooking oil in the air fryer basket and place it in the inner pot of the air fryer.

Place the salmon cakes in the basket and spray some cooking on it.

Close the crisp cover. In the bake mode, set the temperature at 400°f and set the timer to 12 minutes.

Press start to begin the baking. Open the crisp cover, halfway through the cooking and flip the salmon cake and spritz some more oil. Close the lid, so that the instant pot can resume cooking automatically.

Serve hot, along with your favorite touching.

Nutrition:

calories 23

Carbs 12g

Fat 16g

Protein 42g

274) Air fried fish and chips

Preparation time: 15 minutes

cooking: 30 minutes

servings: 4

Ingredients:

6 ounces (4 nos.) Tilapia fillets, skinless

13 ounces (2 nos.) Russet potatoes, scrubbed

1 cup panko breadcrumbs, whole-wheat

½ cup of malt vinegar

2 eggs, large

1 cup all-purpose flour

2 tablespoons water

1¼ teaspoons salt, divided

Vegetable cooking oil spray

Directions:

Scrub wash the potatoes and pat dry. Cut the potatoes in spiral shapes.

Spritz some cooking oil in the air fryer basket and place the potato chips in the air fryer basket.

Put the air fryer basket in the inner pot of the instant pot air fryer. Spray some cooking oil on the chips and close the crisp cover. In the air fry mode, set the temperature at 375 ° f and timer for 10 minutes.

Press start to begin cooking.

Halfway through the cooking, open the crisp lid and shake the air fryer basket for even cooking.

Spry some more cooking oil and close the crisp lid to resume cooking. Once the cooking is over, season it with salt.

In the meantime, using a medium bowl, combine flour and salt.

Whisk the eggs and water in a shallow dish in the meantime.

Mix the panko breadcrumbs and ½ teaspoon salt in the third shallow dish.

Cut the fillets in long strips and dredge them in the flour mix, then dip in the egg mix and lastly dredge in the panko breadcrumbs. Press the coating gently, so that the coating can hold in the fish strips firmly.

Spritz some cooking oil in the air fryer basket and place the coated fillets in the air fryer basket.

Place the air fryer basket in the inner pot of the instant pot air fryer.

Spray some cooking oil on the fillets.

Close the crisp lid.

In the air fry mode, set the temperature at 375 ° f and timer to 10 minutes.

Press start to begin cooking.

Do not overcrowd the air fryer basket, cook it in batches.

Halfway through the cooking, open the crisp cover and flip the fillet chips.

Spray some cooking oil if required.

Close the crisp lid, so that it can resume cooking from where you have stopped.

After cooking, serve hot with an equal portion of potatoes with 2 tablespoons of malt vinegar as dipping.

Nutrition:
calories 415

Carbohydrates: 46g

Fat 7g, protein: 44g

Sodium: 754mg

Sugars: 2g

Saturated fat: 2g

Calcium: 21.3mg

275) Plantain chips in the air fryer

Preparation time: 5 minutes

cooking: 15 minutes

servings:2

Ingredients:

9¾ ounces (1 no.) Green plantain

½ teaspoon of sea salt

Canola oil spray Directions:

Peel and cut the plantain into round slices, make sure to keep them very thin in thickness.

Spray some cooking oil in the air fryer basket and place the plantain slices into it.

Spritz some cooking oil on the plantain slices.

Sprinkle some sea salt Place the air fryer basket in the inner pot of the instant pot air fryer.

Close the crisp lid.

In the air fry mode, select the temperature at 350° f and timer for 18 minutes.

Press start to begin the cooking. Halfway through the cooking, open the crisp lid and shake the air fryer basket.

Spritz some more cooking   oil
        if required.

To prevent burning, keep checking the slices every 5 minutes.

Close the crisp lid to resume the cooking. You don't have to worry about its cooking setting, as the appliance can remember the last cooking option and resume cooking from the point where you have interrupted the cooking.

When cooked, shake the basket and empty the slices in a plate using tongs.

Serve with your favorite condiment.

Nutrition:

calories 415

Carbohydrates: 46g

Fat 7g, protein: 44g

Sodium: 754mg

Sugars: 2g

Saturated fat: 2g

Calcium: 21.3mg

276) Air fried zucchini fried

Preparation time: 10 minutes

cooking: 15 minutes

Servings: 4

Ingredients:

Ounces (2 nos.) Zucchinis, medium size.
½ teaspoon italian seasoning

1 teaspoon onion powder

1 teaspoon garlic powder

1 tablespoon yeast

¼ cup coconut flour

¼ teaspoon pepper

½ teaspoon salt Directions:

Wash, dry and cut the zucchinis into ½ inch thick wedges.

In a large mixing bowl, combine the coconut flour, garlic powder, yeast, onion powder, salt, and pepper with italian seasoning.

Toss the zucchini pieces in the flour mix to coat them evenly.

Transfer the zucchini in the air fryer basket and place them in a layer without overlapping.

Place the air fryer basket in the inner pot of the instant pot air fryer.

Close the crisp lid.

Set the air fryer at 400°f for 15 minutes, under the air fry mode.

Press start to begin the cooking.

Halfway through the cooking, open the crisp lid, and shake the basket for even cooking.

After shaking, close the crisp lid to resume the cooking for the remaining period.

Once the cooking is over, serve it hot.

Nutrition:

calories 33

Carbohydrates: 46g

Fat 7g, protein: 44g

Sodium: 754mg

Sugars: 2g

Saturated fat: 2g

Calcium: 21.3mg

277) Air fried blooming onion

Preparation time: 15 minutes

cooking: 30 minutes

serving: 6

Ingredients:

4½ ounces (1 no.) Yellow onion, large

1 teaspoon onion powder

1 teaspoon garlic powder

2 teaspoons paprika

1 cup breadcrumbs

3 eggs, large

1 teaspoon kosher salt

For the sauce:

3 cups of mayonnaise

¼ teaspoon oregano, dried

½ teaspoon garlic powder

½ teaspoon paprika

1 teaspoon horseradish

2 tablespoons ketchup

1 teaspoon kosher salt   Directions:

Let us begin beating the eggs with 1 teaspoon of water in a shallow bowl. Combine spices, salt, and breadcrumbs in another shallow bowl.

Cut the onion sideways for the shape desired and dip them in the egg wash and then in the breadcrumb mix. Press it down gently for even coating. Place the onion in the air fryer basket and put the air fryer basket in the inner pot of the instant pot air fryer.
Close the crisp lid.
Set the temperature at 375° f under the air fry mode and select the timer for 20 minutes.

Press the start and let the onion cook. In the meantime, prepare the sauce by adding all the sauce ingredients in another bowl.

Serve the onion with a little seasoning of salt and serve it hot with the sauce.

Nutrition: calories

125

Carbohydrates: 46g Fat

7g, protein: 44g

Sodium: 754mg

Sugars: 2g

Saturated fat: 2g

Calcium: 21.3mg

278) Apple chips in instant pot air fryer

Preparation time: 5 minutes

cooking: 20 minutes

servings: 2

Ingredients:

16 ounces (2 nos.) Apple,

large 2 teaspoons sugar ½

teaspoon ground cinnamon

Directions:

Wash, dry apple, and thinly slice. Mix the apple pieces with sugar and cinnamon in a large bowl. Place the coated apple slices in the air fryer basket without overlapping. Put the air fryer basket in the inner pot of the instant pot air fryer.

Close the crisp lid.

Set the temperature at 350°f and timer for 12 minutes in the roast mode.

Press start to begin the roasting.

Halfway through the roasting, open the crisp lid and shake the air fryer basket for even cooking.

Close the crisp lid to resume the roasting.

Keep checking in between to confirm the desired crisp.

Note – the apple slices will continue to crisp as they cool down.

Nutritional values nutrition per serving:

Calories: 129, calories from fat: 3, total fat: 0.4g, saturated fat: 0.1g, trans fat: 0g, trans fat: 0g, cholesterol: 0mg, sodium: 2mg, total carbs: 34g, dietary fiber: 6g, sugars: 26g, protein: 1g

279) Air fried parmesan tortellini

Preparation time: 5 minutes

cooking: 25 minutes

serving: 6

Ingredients:

9-oz tortellini cheese

½ cup parmesan, freshly grated

1 cup panko breadcrumbs

2 eggs, large

1 cup all-purpose flour

1 teaspoon ground black pepper

1 teaspoon kosher salt

½ teaspoon red pepper flakes, crushed

½ teaspoon garlic powder

1 teaspoon oregano, dried Directions:

Cook the tortellini in boiling saltwater, as per the packet instruction, and drain it thoroughly.

In a medium bowl, combine the salt, pepper, red pepper flakes, garlic powder, oregano, parmesan, and panko breadcrumbs.

Whisk the eggs in a shallow bowl. Place the all-purpose flour in a medium shallow bowl.

Dredge the tortellini in the all-purpose flour.

After that, dip in the beaten eggs. Shake off the excess liquid.

Finally, dredge tortellini in the panko mixture. Follow the process for all the tortellini.

Place the coated tortellini in the air fryer basket and put the air fryer basket in the inner pot of instant pot air fryer. Set the temperature at 370° f in the air fry mode and keep the timer for 10 minutes.

Press start to begin the cooking.

Midway through the cooking, open the crisp lid and flip the tortellini.

Close the crisp cover to resume the cooking.

Serve it hot when done.

Nutritional: calories: 262

Calories from fat: 100

Total fat: 11.3g

Saturated at: 6.5g

Trans fat: 0g

Cholesterol: 86mg

Sodium: 1188mg

Total carbs: 26g

Dietary fiber: 1g

Sugars: 4g

Protein: 13g

280) Air fried french toast sticks

Preparation time: 5 minutes

cooking: 8 minutes

servings: 6

Ingredients:

6 slices white wheat bread

½ teaspoon vanilla extract

¼ teaspoon ground cinnamon

3 tablespoons sugar, granulated

⅓ cup whole milk

⅓ cup heavy cream

2 eggs, large

¼ cup maple syrup, to serve

2 tablespoons melted butter Directions:

Combine the eggs, vanilla, cinnamon, sugar, milk, and cream in a large bowl with a pinch of salt.

Coat the mixture on the bread slices.

Brush butter in the bottom of the air fryer basket.

Put it in the inner pot of the instant pot air fryer.

Place the coated bread slices in the air fryer basket without overlapping.

Brush butter on it slightly.

Close the crisp lid.

In the bake mode, set the temperature at 375°f and set the timer for 8 minutes.

Press start to begin the baking. Halfway through the cooking, open the crisp lid and flip the slices.

Close the lid to resume the cooking.

Serve it hot with some maple syrup drizzled on top.

Nutritional: calories: 262

Calories from fat: 100

Total fat: 11.3g

Saturated at: 6.5g

Trans fat: 0g

Cholesterol: 86mg

Sodium: 1188mg

Total carbs: 26g

Dietary fiber: 1g

Sugars: 4g

Protein: 13g

281) Lemon pepper broccoli crunch

Preparation time: 5 minutes

Cooking time: 6 hours

Servings: 4

Ingredients

4cups broccoli florets, chopped into bite sized pieces

1tbsp olive oil

1tsp sea salt

1tsp lemon pepper seasoning

Directions:

Preheat your air fryer to 135 degrees f.

Wash and drain the broccoli florets.

Place the broccoli in a large bowl and toss with the olive oil and sea salt.

Add the broccoli to the basket of your air fryer or spread them in a flat layer on the tray of your air fryer (either option will work!).

Cook in the air fryer for about 6 hours, tossing the broccoli every hour or so to cook evenly. Essentially, you will be dehydrating the broccoli.

Once the broccoli is fully dried, remove it from the air fryer, toss with the lemon pepper seasoning, and then let cool. It will keep crisping as it cools.

Enjoy fresh or store in an airtight container for up to a month.

Nutritional: calories: 53

Calories from fat: 53

Total fat: 11.3g

Saturated at: 6.5g

Trans fat: 0g

Cholesterol: 86mg

Sodium: 1188mg

Total carbs: 26g
Dietary fiber: 1g

Sugars: 4g

Protein: 13g

282) Sweet broccoli crunch

Preparation time: 5 minutes

Cooking time: 6 hours

Servings: 4

Ingredients

4cups broccoli florets, chopped into bite sized pieces

1tbsp olive oil

1tsp sea salt

1tsp granulated erythritol Directions:

Preheat your air fryer to 135 degrees f. Wash and drain the broccoli florets.

Place the broccoli in a large bowl and toss with the olive oil, erythritol, and sea salt.

Add the broccoli to the basket of your air fryer or spread them in a flat layer on the tray of your air fryer (either option will work!).

Cook in the air fryer for about 6 hours, tossing the broccoli every hour or so to cook evenly. Essentially, you will be dehydrating the broccoli.

Once the broccoli is fully dried, remove it from the air fryer and then let cool. It will keep crisping as it cools.

Enjoy fresh or store in an airtight container for up to a month.

Nutritional: calories: 262

Calories from fat: 100

Total fat: 11.3g

Saturated at: 6.5g

Trans fat: 0g

Cholesterol: 86mg

Sodium: 1188mg

Total carbs: 26g

Dietary fiber: 1g

Sugars: 4g

Protein: 13g

283) Maple broccoli crunch

Preparation time: 5 minutes

Cooking time: 6 hours

Servings: 4

Ingredients

4cups broccoli florets, chopped into bite sized pieces

1tbsp olive oil

1tsp sea salt

1½ tsp maple extract   Directions:

Preheat your air fryer to 135 degrees f. Wash and drain the broccoli florets.

Place the broccoli in a large bowl and toss with the olive oil, maple extract, and sea salt.

Add the broccoli to the basket of your air fryer or spread them in a flat layer on

the tray of your air fryer (either option will work!).

Cook in the air fryer for about 6 hours, tossing the broccoli every hour or so to cook evenly. Essentially, you will be dehydrating the broccoli.

Once the broccoli is fully dried, remove it from the air fryer and then let cool. It will keep crisping as it cools.

Enjoy fresh or store in an airtight container for up to a month.

Nutritional: calories: 54

Calories from fat: 51

Total fat: 11.3g

Saturated at: 6.5g

Trans fat: 0g

Cholesterol: 86mg

Sodium: 1188mg

Total carbs: 26g

Dietary fiber: 1g

Sugars: 4g

Protein: 13g

Cook in the air fryer for about 6 hours, tossing the florets every hour or so to cook evenly. Essentially, you will be dehydrating the veggies.

Once the florets are fully dried, remove it from the air fryer and then let cool. It will keep crisping as it cools.

Enjoy fresh or store in an airtight container for up to a month.

Nutritional: calories: 53

Calories from fat: 51

Total fat: 11.3g

Saturated at: 6.5g

Trans fat: 0g

Cholesterol: 86mg

Sodium: 1188mg

Total carbs: 26g

Dietary fiber: 1g

Sugars: 4g

Protein: 13g

284) Veggie crunch

Preparation time: 5 minutes

Cooking time: 6 hours

Servings: 4

Ingredients

2cups broccoli florets, chopped into bite sized pieces

2cups cauliflower florets, chopped into bite sized pieces   1tbsp olive oil

1tsp sea salt   Directions:

Preheat your air fryer to 135 degrees f. Wash and drain the florets.

Place the florets in a large bowl and toss with the olive oil and sea salt.

Add the florets to the basket of your air fryer or spread them in a flat layer on the tray of your air fryer (either option will work!).

285) Chili lime broccoli crunch

Preparation time: 5 minutes

Cooking time: 6 hours

Servings: 4

Ingredients

4cups broccoli florets, chopped into bite sized pieces

1tbsp olive oil

1tsp sea salt

1tsp lime zest

1tbsp lime juice

1tsp chili powder

Directions:

Preheat your air fryer to 135 degrees f. Wash and drain the broccoli florets.

Place the broccoli in a large bowl and toss with the olive oil, lime juice, lime zest and sea salt.

Add the broccoli to the basket of your air fryer or spread them in a flat layer on the tray of your air fryer (either option will work!).

Cook in the air fryer for about 6 hours, tossing the broccoli every hour or so to cook evenly. Essentially, you will be dehydrating the broccoli.

Once the broccoli is fully dried, remove it from the air fryer, toss with the chili powder, and then let cool. It will keep crisping as it cools.

Enjoy fresh or store in an airtight container for up to a month.

Nutritional: calories: 53

Calories from fat: 51

Total fat: 11.3g

Saturated at: 6.5g

Trans fat: 0g

Cholesterol: 86mg

Sodium: 1188mg

Total carbs: 26g

Dietary fiber: 1g

Sugars: 4g

Protein: 13g

286) Zucchini chips

Preparation time: 15 minutes

Cooking time: 4 hours

Servings: 8

Ingredients

4cups very thin zucchini slices

2tbsp olive oil

2tsp sea salt   Directions:

Preheat your air fryer to 135 degrees f.

Toss the thin zucchini slices with the oil and sea salt.

Place the zucchini on the air fryer tray or in the air fryer basket.

Cook for 4 hours, tossing the zucchini occasionally to allow it to dehydrate evenly.

Once crisp, remove the zucchini from the air fryer and enjoy!

Nutritional: calories: 262

Calories from fat: 100

Total fat: 11.3g

Saturated at: 6.5g

Trans fat: 0g

Cholesterol: 86mg

Sodium: 1188mg

Total carbs: 26g

Dietary fiber: 1g

Sugars: 4g

Protein: 13g

287) Cayenne zucchini chips

Preparation time: 15 minutes

Cooking time: 4 hours

Servings: 8

Ingredients

4cups very thin zucchini slices

2tbsp olive oil

2tsp sea salt

1tsp cayenne pepper   Directions:

Preheat your air fryer to 135 degrees f.

Toss the thin zucchini slices with the oil, cayenne and sea salt.

Place the zucchini on the air fryer tray or in the air fryer basket.

Cook for 4 hours, tossing the zucchini occasionally to allow it to dehydrate evenly.

Once crisp, remove the zucchini from the air fryer and enjoy!   Nutritional: calories: 42

Calories from fat: 51

Total fat: 11.3g

Saturated at: 6.5g

Trans fat: 0g

Cholesterol: 86mg

Sodium: 1188mg

Total carbs: 26g

Dietary fiber: 1g

Sugars: 4g

Protein: 13g

288) Salt and vinegar zucchini chips

Preparation time: 15 minutes

Cooking time: 4 hours

Servings: 8

Ingredients

4cups very thin zucchini slices

2tbsp olive oil

2tsp sea salt

1tbsp white balsamic vinegar

Directions:

Preheat your air fryer to 135 degrees f.

Toss the thin zucchini slices with the oil, vinegar and sea salt.

Place the zucchini on the air fryer tray or in the air fryer basket.

Cook for 4 hours, tossing the zucchini occasionally to allow it to dehydrate evenly.

Once crisp, remove the zucchini from the air fryer and enjoy!

Nutritional: calories: 32

Calories from fat: 12

Total fat: 11.3g

Saturated at: 6.5g

Trans fat: 0g

Cholesterol: 86mg

Sodium: 1188mg

Total carbs: 26g

Dietary fiber: 1g

Sugars: 4g

Protein: 13g

289) Smoked zucchini chips

Preparation time: 15 minutes

Cooking time: 4 hours

Servings: 8

Ingredients

4cups very thin zucchini slices

2tbsp olive oil

2tsp smoked sea salt   Directions:

Preheat your air fryer to 135 degrees f.
Toss the thin zucchini slices with the oil and smoked sea salt.

Place the zucchini on the air fryer tray or in the air fryer basket.

Cook for 4 hours, tossing the zucchini occasionally to allow it to dehydrate evenly.

Once crisp, remove the zucchini from the air fryer and enjoy!

Nutritional: calories: 262

Calories from fat: 100

Total fat: 11.3g

Saturated at: 6.5g

Trans fat: 0g

Cholesterol: 86mg

Sodium: 1188mg

Total carbs: 26g

Dietary fiber: 1g

Sugars: 4g

Protein: 13g

290) Yellow zucchini chips

Preparation time: 15 minutes

Cooking time: 4 hours

Servings: 8

Ingredients

4cups very thin yellow zucchini slices

2tbsp olive oil

2tsp sea salt   Directions:

Preheat your air fryer to 135 degrees f.

Toss the thin zucchini slices with the oil and sea salt. Place the zucchini on the air fryer tray or in the air fryer basket.

Cook for 4 hours, tossing the zucchini occasionally to allow it to dehydrate evenly. Once crisp, remove the zucchini from the air fryer and enjoy!

Nutritional: calories: 262 Calories from fat: 100 Total fat: 11.3g

Saturated at: 6.5g Trans fat: 0g

Cholesterol: 86mg Sodium: 1188mg

Total carbs: 26g Dietary fiber: 1g

Sugars: 4g Protein: 13g

291) Soft pretzels

Preparation time: 15 minutes

Cooking time: 14 minutes

Servings: 6

Ingredients

2cups almond flour

1tbsp baking powder

1tsp garlic powder

1tsp onion powder

3eggs

5tbsp softened cream cheese

3cups mozzarella cheese, grated

1tsp sea salt   Directions:

Preheat your air fryer to 400 degrees f and prepare the air fryer tray with parchment paper. Place the almond flour, onion powder, baking powder and garlic powder in a large bowl and stir well.

Combine the cream cheese and mozzarella in a separate bowl and melt in the microwave, heating slowly and stirring several times to ensure the cheese melts and does not burn.

Add two eggs to the almond flour mix along with the melted cheese. Stir well until a dough form.

Divide the dough into six equal pieces and roll into your desired pretzel shape.

Place the pretzels on the prepared sheet tray.

Whisk the remaining eggs and brush over the pretzels then sprinkle them all with the sea salt.

Bake in the air fryer for 12 minutes or until the pretzels are golden brown.

Remove from the air fryer and enjoy while warm!

Nutritional: calories: 422

Calories from fat: 100 Total fat: 11.3g

Saturated at: 6.5g Trans fat: 0g

Cholesterol: 86mg Sodium: 1188mg

Total carbs: 26g Dietary fiber: 1g

Sugars: 4g

Protein: 13g

292) Soft garlic parmesan pretzels

Preparation time: 15 minutes

Cooking time: 14 minutes

Servings: 6

Ingredients

2cups almond flour

1tbsp baking powder

1tsp garlic powder

1tsp onion powder

3eggs

5tbsp softened cream cheese

3cups mozzarella cheese, grated

1tsp sea salt

½ tsp garlic powder

¼ cup parmesan cheese Directions:

Preheat your air fryer to 400 degrees f and prepare the air fryer tray with parchment paper.

Place the almond flour, onion powder, baking powder and 1 tsp garlic powder in a large bowl and stir well.

Combine the cream cheese and mozzarella in a separate bowl and melt in the microwave, heating slowly and stirring several times to ensure the cheese melts and does not burn.

Add two eggs to the almond flour mix along with the melted cheese. Stir well until a dough form.

Divide the dough into six equal pieces and roll into your desired pretzel shape.

Place the pretzels on the prepared sheet tray.

Whisk the remaining eggs and brush over the pretzels then sprinkle them all with the sea salt, parmesan, and ½ tsp garlic powder.

Bake in the air fryer for 12 minutes or until the pretzels are golden brown.

Cholesterol: 86mg

Sodium: 1188mg parchment paper.
Total carbs: 26g

Dietary fiber: 1g and salt in a large bowl and stir well.

Sugars: 4g

Protein: 13g

293) Soft cinnamon pretzels

Preparation time: 15 minutes
Cooking time: 14 minutes

Servings: 6

Ingredients

2cups almond flour

1tbsp baking powder

Remove from the air fryer and enjoy while warm!

Nutritional: calories: 452

Calories from fat: 100

Total fat: 11.3g

Saturated at: 6.5g

Trans fat: 0g

Preheat your air fryer to 400 degrees f and prepare the air fryer tray with

Place the almond flour, baking powder

Combine the cream cheese and mozzarella in a separate bowl and melt in the microwave, heating slowly and stirring several times to ensure the cheese melts and does not burn.

Add two eggs to the almond flour mix along with the melted cheese. Stir well until a dough form.

Divide the dough into six equal pieces and roll into your desired pretzel shape.

Place the pretzels on the prepared sheet tray.

1tsp salt
3eggs
5tbsp softened cream cheese

3cups mozzarella cheese, grated
½ tsp ground cinnamon

Directions:

Total fat: 11.3g

Saturated at: 6.5g

Trans fat: 0g

Cholesterol: 86mg

Sodium: 1188mg

Total carbs: 26g

Dietary fiber: 1g

Sugars: 4g

Protein: 13g

294) Soft pecan pretzels

Preparation time: 15 minutes

Cooking time: 14 minutes

Servings: 6

Whisk the remaining eggs and brush over the pretzels then sprinkle them all with the cinnamon.

Bake in the air fryer for 12 minutes or until the pretzels are golden brown.

Remove from the air fryer and enjoy while warm!

Nutritional: calories: 432

Calories from fat: 100
Ingredients

2cups almond flour

1tbsp baking powder

1tsp garlic powder

1tsp onion powder

3eggs

5tbsp softened cream cheese

3cups mozzarella cheese, grated   1tsp sea salt

¼ cup chopped pecans   Directions:

Preheat your air fryer to 400 degrees f and prepare the air fryer tray with parchment paper.

Place the almond flour, onion powder, baking powder and garlic powder in a large bowl and stir well.

Combine the cream cheese and mozzarella in a separate bowl and melt in the microwave, heating slowly and stirring several times to ensure the cheese melts and does not burn.

Add two eggs to the almond flour mix along with the melted cheese. Stir well until a dough form.

Divide the dough into six equal pieces and roll into your desired pretzel shape.

Place the pretzels on the prepared sheet tray.

Whisk the remaining eggs and brush over the pretzels then sprinkle them all with the sea salt and chopped pecans

Bake in the air fryer for 12 minutes or until the pretzels are golden brown.

Remove from the air fryer and enjoy while warm!

Nutritional: calories: 512

Calories from fat: 100

Total fat: 11.3g

Saturated at: 6.5g

Trans fat: 0g

Cholesterol: 86mg

Sodium: 1188mg

Total carbs: 26g

Dietary fiber: 1g

Sugars: 4g

Protein: 13g

295) Soft cheesy pretzels

Preparation time: 15 minutes

Cooking time: 14 minutes

Servings: 6

Ingredients

2cups almond flour

1tbsp baking powder

1tbsp grated parmesan cheese

1tsp garlic powder

3eggs

5tbsp softened cream cheese

3cups mozzarella cheese, grated

1tsp sea salt

½ grated cheddar cheese

Directions:

Preheat your air fryer to 400 degrees f and prepare the air fryer tray with parchment paper.

Place the almond flour, parmesan, baking powder and garlic powder in a large bowl and stir well.

Combine the cream cheese and mozzarella in a separate bowl and melt in the microwave, heating slowly and stirring several times to ensure the cheese melts and does not burn.

Add two eggs to the almond flour mix along with the melted cheese. Stir well until a dough form.

Divide the dough into six equal pieces and roll into your desired pretzel shape.

Place the pretzels on the prepared sheet tray.

Whisk the remaining eggs and brush over the pretzels then sprinkle them all with the sea salt and the grated cheddar cheese.

Bake in the air fryer for 12 minutes or until the pretzels are golden brown.

Remove from the air fryer and enjoy while warm!

Nutritional: calories: 513

Calories from fat: 100

Total fat: 11.3g

Saturated at: 6.5g

Trans fat: 0g

Cholesterol: 86mg

Sodium: 1188mg

Total carbs: 26g

Dietary fiber: 1g

Sugars: 4g

Protein: 13g

296) Sweet zucchini chips

Preparation time: 15 minutes

Cooking time: 4 hours

Servings: 8

Ingredients

4cups very thin zucchini slices

2tbsp olive oil

2tsp sea salt

1tbsp   granulated   erythritol

Directions:

Preheat your air fryer to 135 degrees f.

Toss the thin zucchini slices with the oil, erythritol and sea salt.

Place the zucchini on the air fryer tray or in the air fryer basket.

Cook for 4 hours, tossing the zucchini occasionally to allow it to dehydrate evenly.

Once crisp, remove the zucchini from the air fryer and enjoy!

Nutritional: calories: 40

Calories from fat: 12

Total fat: 11.3g

Saturated at: 6.5g

Trans fat: 0g

Cholesterol: 86mg

Sodium: 1188mg

Total carbs: 26g

Dietary fiber: 1g

Sugars: 4g

Protein: 13g

297) Cucumber chips

Preparation time: 15 minutes

Cooking time: 3 hours

Servings: 4

Ingredients

4cups very thin cucumber slices

2tbsp apple cider vinegar

2tsp sea salt   Directions:

Preheat your air fryer to 200 degrees f.

Place the cucumber slices on a paper towel and layer another paper towel on top to absorb the moisture in the cucumbers.

Place the dried slices in a large bowl and toss with the vinegar and salt.

Place the cucumber slices on a tray lined with parchment and then bake in the air fryer for 3 hours. The cucumbers will begin to curl and brown slightly.

Turn off the air fryer and let the cucumber slices cool inside the fryer (this will help them dry a little more).

Enjoy right away or store in an airtight container.

Nutritional: calories: 15

Calories from fat: 11

Total fat: 8.3g

Saturated at: 6.5g

Trans fat: 0g

Cholesterol: 86mg

Sodium: 1188mg

Total carbs: 26g

Dietary fiber: 1g

Sugars: 4g

Protein: 13g

Vegetarian

298) Homemade french fries

Preparation time: 30 minutes

Cooking time: 28 minutes servings: 4

Ingredients:

2 reddish potatoes, cut into strips of 76 x 25 mm

1 liter of cold water, to soak the potatoes

15 ml of oil

3g garlic powder

2g of paprika

Salt and pepper to taste Tomato sauce or ranch sauce, to serve Direction:

Cut the potatoes into 76 x 25 mm strips and soak them in water for 15 minutes.

Drain the potatoes, rinse with cold, dry water with paper towels.

Add oil and spices to the potatoes, until they are completely covered.

Preheat the air fryer, set it to 195°c.

Add the potatoes to the preheated air fryer. Set the timer to 28 minutes.

Be sure to shake the baskets in the middle of cooking.

Remove the baskets from the air fryer when you have finished cooking and season the fries with salt and pepper.

Serve with tomato sauce or ranch sauce.

Nutrition: calories: 390

Fat: 36g

Carbohydrates: 42g

Protein: 5g

Sugar: 4g

Cholesterol: 0mg

299) Sweet potato chips

Preparation time: 5 minutes

Cooking time: 10 minutes.

Servings: 4

Ingredients:

2 large sweet potatoes, cut into strips 25 mm thick

15 ml of oil

10g of salt

2g black pepper

2g of paprika

2g garlic powder   2g onion powder

Direction:

Cut the sweet potatoes into strips 25 mm thick.

Preheat the air fryer for a few minutes.

Add the cut sweet potatoes in a large bowl and mix with the oil until the potatoes are all evenly coated.

Sprinkle salt, black pepper, paprika, garlic powder and onion powder. Mix well.

Place the french fries in the preheated baskets and cook for 10 minutes at 205°c. Be sure to shake the baskets halfway through cooking.

Nutrition: calories: 130

Fat: 0g

Carbohydrates: 29g

Protein: 2g

Sugar: 9g

Cholesterol: 0mg

300) Cajun style french fries

Preparation time: 30 minutes

Cooking time: 28 minutes.

Servings: 4

Ingredients:

2 reddish potatoes, peeled and cut into strips of 76 x 25 mm 1 liter of cold water

15 ml of oil

7g of cajun seasoning

1g cayenne pepper

Tomato sauce or ranch sauce, to serve Direction:

Cut the potatoes into 76 x 25 mm strips and soak them in water for 15 minutes. Drain the potatoes, rinse with cold, dry water with paper towels. Preheat the air fryer, set it to 195°c.

Add oil and spices to the potatoes, until they are completely covered.

Add the potatoes to the preheated air fryer and set the timer to 28 minutes.

Be sure to shake the baskets in the middle of cooking   Remove the baskets from the air fryer when you have finished cooking and season the fries with salt and pepper.

Serve with tomato sauce or ranch sauce.

Nutrition: calories: 156

Fat: 8.01g Carbohydrate: 20.33g

Protein: 1.98g Sugar: 0.33g

Cholesterol: 0mg

301) Fried zucchini

Preparation time: 10 minutes.

Cooking time: 8 minutes.

Servings: 4

Ingredients:

2 medium zucchinis, cut into strips 19 mm thick

60g all-purpose flour

12g of salt

2g black pepper

2 beaten eggs

15 ml of milk

84g italian seasoned breadcrumbs

25g grated parmesan cheese

Nonstick spray oil

Ranch sauce, to

serve

Direction:

Cut the zucchini into strips 19 mm thick.

Mix with the flour, salt, and pepper on a plate. Mix the eggs and milk in a separate dish. Put breadcrumbs and parmesan cheese in another dish.

Cover each piece of zucchini with flour, then dip them in egg and pass them through the crumbs. Leave aside.

Preheat the air fryer, set it to 175°c.

Place the covered zucchini in the preheated air fryer and spray with oil spray. Set the timer to 8 minutes and press start pause.

Be sure to shake the baskets in the middle of cooking.

Serve with tomato sauce or ranch sauce.

Nutrition: calories: 67

Fat: 4.1g

Carbohydrates: 4.5g

Protein: 3.3g

Sugar: 1.47g

Cholesterol: 20.7mg

302) Fried avocado

Preparation time: 15 minutes.

Cooking time: 10 minutes.

Servings: 2

Ingredients:

2 avocados cut into wedges 25 mm thick

50g pan crumbs bread

2g garlic powder

2g onion powder

1g smoked paprika

1g cayenne pepper

Salt and pepper to taste

60g all-purpose flour

2 eggs, beaten

Nonstick spray oil

Tomato sauce or ranch sauce, to serve Direction:

Cut the avocados into 25 mm thick pieces.

Combine the crumbs, garlic powder, onion powder, smoked paprika, cayenne pepper and salt in a bowl.

Separate each wedge of avocado in the flour, then dip the beaten eggs and stir in the breadcrumb mixture.

Preheat the air fryer.

Place the avocados in the preheated air fryer baskets, spray with oil spray and cook at 205°c for 10 minutes. Turn the fried avocado halfway through cooking and sprinkle with cooking oil.

Serve with tomato sauce or ranch sauce.

Nutrition: calories: 96

Fat: 8.8g

Carbohydrates: 5.12g

Protein: 1.2g

Sugar: 0.4g

Cholesterol: 0mg

303) Vegetables in air fryer

Preparation time: 20 minutes.

Cooking time: 30 minutes.

Servings: 2

Ingredients:

2 potatoes

1 zucchini

1 onion

1 red pepper

1 green pepper

Direction:

Cut the potatoes into slices.

Cut the onion into rings.

Cut the zucchini slices

Cut the peppers into strips.

Put all the ingredients in the bowl and add a little salt, ground pepper and some extra virgin olive oil.

Mix well.

Pass to the basket of the air fryer.

Select 1600c, 30 minutes.

Check that the vegetables are to your liking.

Nutrition: calories: 135

Fat: 11g

Carbohydrates: 8g

Protein: 1g

Sugar: 2g

Cholesterol: 0mg

304) Crispy rye bread snacks with guacamole and anchovies

Preparation time: 10 minutes.

Cooking time: 10 minutes.

Servings: 4

Ingredients:

4 slices of rye bread

Guacamole

Anchovies in oil Direction:

Cut each slice of bread into 3 strips of bread.

Place in the basket of the air fryer, without piling up, and we go in batches giving it the touch you want to give it. You can select 1800c, 10 minutes.

When you have all the crusty rye bread strips, put a layer of guacamole on top, whether homemade or commercial.

In each bread, place 2 anchovies on the guacamole.

Nutrition: calories: 180

Fat: 11.6g

Carbohydrates: 16g

Protein: 6.2g

Sugar: 0g

Cholesterol: 19.6mg

305) Mushrooms stuffed with tomato

Preparation time: 5 minutes.

Cooking time: 50 minutes.

Servings: 4

Ingredients:

8 large mushrooms

250g of minced meat

4 cloves of garlic

Extra virgin olive oil

Salt

Ground pepper

Flour, beaten egg and breadcrumbs

Frying oil

Fried tomato sauce

Direction:

Remove the stem from the mushrooms and chop it. Peel the garlic and chop. Put some extra virgin olive oil in a pan and add the garlic and mushroom stems.

Sauté and add the minced meat. Sauté well until the meat is well cooked and season.

Fill the mushrooms with the minced meat.

Press well and take the freezer for 30 minutes.

Pass the mushrooms with flour, beaten egg and breadcrumbs. Beaten egg and breadcrumbs.

Place the mushrooms in the basket of the air fryer.

Select 20 minutes, 1800c.

Distribute the mushrooms once cooked in the dishes.

Heat the tomato sauce and cover the stuffed mushrooms.

Nutrition: calories: 160

Fat: 7.96g

Carbohydrates: 19.41g

Protein: 7.94g

Sugar: 9.19g

Cholesterol: 0mg

306) Spiced potato wedges

Preparation time: 15.

Cooking time: 40 minutes.

Serve 4

Ingredients:

8 medium potatoes

Salt

Ground pepper

Garlic powder

Aromatic herbs, the one we like the most

2 tbsp extra virgin olive oil 4 tbsp breadcrumbs or chickpea flour

Direction:

Put the unpeeled potatoes in a pot with boiling water and a little salt.

Let cook 5 minutes. Drain and let cool. Cut into thick segments, without peeling.

Put the potatoes in a bowl and add salt, pepper, garlic powder, the aromatic herb that we have chosen oil and breadcrumbs or chickpea flour.

Stir well and leave 15 minutes. Pass to the basket of the air fryer and select 20 minutes, 1800c.

From time to time shake the basket so that the potatoes mix and change position. Check that they are tender.

Nutrition: calories: 121

Fat: 3g

Carbohydrates: 19g

Protein: 2g

Sugar: 0g

Cholesterol: 0mg

307) Egg stuffed zucchini balls

Preparation time: 15 minutes.

Cooking time: 45-60 minutes.

Servings: 4

Ingredients:

2 zucchinis

1 onion

1 egg

120g of grated cheese

4 eggs

Salt

Ground pepper

Flour

Direction:

Chop the zucchini and onion in the thermomix, 10 seconds speed 8, in the cuisine with the kneader chopper at speed 10 about 15 seconds or we can chop the onion by hand and the zucchini grate. No matter how you do it, the important thing is that the zucchini and onion are as small as possible.

Put in a bowl and add the cheese and the egg. Pepper and bind well.

Incorporate the flour, until you have a very brown dough with which you can wrap the eggs without problems.

Cook the eggs and peel.

Cover the eggs with the zucchini dough and pass through the flour.

Place the four balls in the basket of the air fryer and paint with oil.

Select 1800c and leave for 45 to 60 minutes or until you see that the balls are crispy on the outside.

Serve over a layer of mayonnaise or aioli.

Nutrition: calories: 23

Fat: 0.5g

Carbohydrates: 2g

Protein: 1.8g

Sugar: 0g

Cholesterol: 15mg

308) Vegetables with provolone

Preparation time: 10 minutes.

Cooking time: 30 minutes.

Servings: 4

Ingredients:

1 bag of 400g of frozen tempura vegetables

Extra virgin olive oil

Salt

1 slice of provolone cheese

Direction:

Put the vegetables in the basket of the air fryer. Add some strands of extra virgin olive oil and close.

Select 20 minutes, 2000c.

Pass the vegetables to a clay pot and place the provolone cheese on top.

Take to the oven, 1800c, about 10 minutes or so or until you see that the cheese has melted to your liking.

Nutrition: calories: 104

Fat: 8g

Carbohydrates: 0g

Protein: 8g

Sugar: 0g

Cholesterol: 0mg

309) Spicy potatoes

Preparation time: 10 minutes.

Cooking time: 30 minutes.

Servings: 4

Ingredients:

400g potatoes

2 tbsp spicy paprika

1 tbsp olive oil

Caspary or cottage cheese

Salt to taste

Direction:

Wash the potatoes with a brush. Unpeeled, cut vertically in a crescent shape, about 1 finger thick place the potatoes in a bowl and cover with water. Let stand for about half an hour.

Preheat the air fryer. Set the timer of 5 minutes and the temperature to 2000c.

Drain the water from the potatoes and dry with paper towels or a clean cloth. Put them back in the bowl and pour the oil, salt and paprika over them. Mix well with your hands so that all of them are covered evenly with the spice mixture. Pour the spiced potatoes in the basket of the air fryer. Set the timer for 30 minutes and press the power button. Stir the potatoes in half the time.

Remove the potatoes from the air fryer, place on a plate.

Serve with cheese and sauce.

Nutrition: calories: 153

Fat: 4g

Carbohydrates: 26

Protein: 3g

Sugar: 0g

Cholesterol: 5mg

310) Scrambled eggs with beans, zucchini, potatoes and onions

Preparation time: 30 minutes.

Cooking time: 35 minutes.

Servings: 4

Ingredients:

300g of beans

2 onions

1 zucchini

4 potatoes

8 eggs

Extra virgin olive oil

Salt

Ground pepper

A splash of soy

sauce

Direction:

Put the beans taken from their pod to cook in abundant saltwater. Drain when they are tender and reserve.

Peel the potatoes and cut into dice. Season and put some threads of oil. Mix and take to the air fryer. Select 1800c, 15 minutes.

After that time, add together with the potatoes, diced zucchini, and onion in julienne, mix and select 1800c, 20 minutes.

From time to time mix and stir.

Pass the contents of the air fryer together with the beans to a pan.

Add a little soy sauce and salt to taste.

Sauté and peel the eggs.

Do the scrambled.

Nutrition: calories: 65

Fat: 0.4g

Carbohydrates: 8.6g

Proteins: 4.6g

Sugar: 0g

Cholesterol: 0mg

311) French toast

Preparation time: 5 minutes.

Cooking time: 15 minutes.

Servings: 8 Ingredients:

For the bread:

500g of flour

25g of oil

300 g of water

25g of fresh bread yeast

12g of salt

For french toast:

 milk and cinnamon or milk and sweet wine Eggs

Honey

Direction:

The first thing is to make bread a day before. Put in the masterchef gourmet the ingredients of the bread and knead 1 minute at speed 1. Let the dough rise 1 hour and knead 1 minute at speed 1 again. Remove the dough and divide into 4 portions. Make a ball and spread like a pizza. Roll up to make a small loaf of bread and let rise 1 hour or so.

Take to the oven and bake 40 minutes, 2000c. Let the bread cool on a rack and reserve for the next day. Cut the bread into slices and reserve. Prepare the milk to wet the slices of bread. To do so, put the milk to heat, like 500 ml or so with a cinnamon stick or the same milk with a glass of sweet wine, as you like. When the milk has started to boil, remove from heat, and let cool.

Beat the eggs. Place a rack on a plate and we dip the slices of bread in the cold milk, then in the beaten egg and pass to the rack with the plate underneath to release the excess liquid. Put the slices of bread in the bucket of the air fryer, in batches, not piled up, and we take the air fryer, 180 degrees, 10 minutes each batch.

When you have all the slices passed through the air fryer, put the honey in a casserole, like 500g, next to 1 small glass of water and 4 tablespoons of sugar.

When the honey starts to boil, lower the heat, and pass the bread slices through the honey. Place in a fountain and the rest of the honey we put it on top, bathing again the french toast. Ready our french toast, when they cool, they can already be eaten.

Nutrition: calories: 224

Fat: 15.2g

Carbohydrates: 17.39g

Protein: 4.81g

Sugar: 5.76g

Cholesterol: 84mg

312) Sweet potato salt and pepper

Preparation time: 5 minutes.

Cooking time: 20 minutes.

Servings: 4

Ingredients:

1 large sweet potato

Extra virgin olive oil

Salt

Ground pepper

Direction:

Peel the sweet potato and cut into thin strips, if you have a mandolin it will be easier for you.

Wash well and put salt.

Add a little oil to impregnate the sweet potato in strips and place in the air fryer basket.

Select 1800c, 30 minutes or so. From time to time, shake the basket so that the sweet potato moves.

Pass to a tray or plate and sprinkle with fine salt and ground pepper.

Nutrition: calories: 107

Fat: 0.6g

Carbohydrates: 24.19g

Protein: 1.61g

Sugar: 5.95g

Cholesterol: 0mg

313) Potatoes with provencal herbs with cheese

Preparation time: 5 minutes.

Cooking time: 20 minutes.

Servings: 4

Ingredients:

1kg of potatoes

Provencal herbs

Extra virgin olive oil

Salt   Grated

cheese

Direction:

Peel the potatoes and cut the cane salt and sprinkle with provencal herbs.

Put in the basket and add some strands of extra virgin olive oil.

Take the air fryer and select 1800c, 20 minutes.

Take out and move on to a large plate.

Cover cheese.

Gratin in the microwave or in the oven, a few minutes until the cheese is melted.

Nutrition: calories: 437

Fat: 25g

Carbohydrates: 42g

Protein: 9g

Sugar: 0g

Cholesterol: 0mg

314) Potato wedges

Preparation time: 3 minutes.

Cooking time: 20 minutes.

Servings: 4

Ingredients:

2 large thick potatoes, rinsed and cut into wedges 102 mm long

23 ml of olive oil

3g garlic powder

1g onion powder

3g of salt

1g black pepper

5g grated parmesan cheese

Tomato sauce or ranch sauce, for server
Direction:

Cut the potatoes into 102 mm long pieces.

Preheat the air fryer for 5 minutes. Set it to 195°c.

Cover the potatoes with olive oil and mix the condiments and parmesan cheese until they are well covered.

Add the potatoes to the preheated fryer. Set the time to 20 minutes.

Be sure to shake the baskets in the middle of cooking.

Serve with tomato sauce or ranch sauce.

Nutrition: calories: 156

Fat: 8.01g

Carbohydrate: 20.33g

Protein: 1.98g

Sugar: 0.33g

Cholesterol: 0mg

315) Okra fritter chaffe

Preparation time: 10 minutes

Cooking time: 10 minutes

Servings: 2

Ingredients:

Egg: 1

Mozzarella cheese: ¼ cup

Onion powder: ½ tbsp

Heavy cream: 2 tbsp

Mayo: 1 tbsp

Garlic: 2 cloves (finely chopped)

Almond flour: ¼ cup

Okra: 1 cup

Salt: ¼ tsp or as per your taste Black

pepper: ¼ tsp or as per your taste

Directions:

Combine egg, mayo, and heavy cream and whisk

When mixed, add almond flour and make a uniform batter

Leave it for 5-10 minutes

Now add okra and rest of the ingredients and mix well

Preheat a mini waffle maker if needed and grease it

Pour the mixture to the lower plate of the waffle maker and spread it evenly to cover the plate properly   Cook for at least 4 minutes to get the desired crunch

Remove the chaffle from the heat Make as many chaffles as your mixture and waffle maker allow   Serve hot and enjoy!

Nutrition: 258 calories

20.6g fat

6.2g carbs

46.1g protein

2.1g sugars

1.7g fiber

316) Spiced coriander chaffle

Preparation time: 5 minutes

Cooking time: 10 minutes

Servings: 2

Ingredients:

Egg: 1

Cheddar cheese: ½ cup (shredded)

Thyme: 1 tsp

Allspice: a pinch

Salt and pepper: as per your taste

Coriander: ½ cup chopped

Directions:

Mix all the ingredients well together

Pour a layer on a preheated waffle iron

Cook the chaffle for around 5 minutes

Make as many chaffles as your mixture and waffle maker allow

Nutrition: 258 calories

20.6g fat

6.2g carbs

46.1g protein 2.1g sugars

1.7g fiber

317) Pickled spinach chaffles

Preparation time: 15 minutes

Cooking time: 10 minutes

Servings: 2

Ingredients:

Egg: 1

Spinach: ½ cup chopped, boiled, and drained

Cheddar cheese: ½ cup (shredded)

Pork panko: ½ cup Pickle

slices: 6-8 thin Directions:

Mix egg, spinach, cheese, and pork panko well together Pour a thin layer on a preheated waffle iron

Remove any excess juice from pickles Add pickle slices and pour again more mixture over the top
Cook the chaffle for around 5 minutes Make as many chaffles as your mixture and waffle maker allow Nutrition: 258 calories

20.6g fat

6.2g carbs

46.1g protein

2.1g sugars

1.7g fiber

318) Salty zucchini onion chaffles

Preparation time: 5 minutes
Cooking time: 10 minutes
Servings: 2

Ingredients:

Egg: 1

Mozzarella cheese: 1/2 cup (shredded)

Zucchini: ½ cup finely grated

Onion: ½ cup chopped

Garlic powder: ½ tsp

Pepper: ¼ tsp

Salt: ¼ tsp

Directions:

Preheat a mini waffle maker if needed and grease it

In a mixing bowl, add all the ingredients of the chaffle and mix well
Pour the mixture to the waffle maker
Cook for at least 4 minutes to get the desired crunch and make as many chaffles as your batter allows
Nutrition: 258 calories

20.6g fat

6.2g carbs

46.1g protein

2.1g sugars

1.7g fiber

319) Minty chaffle salad bowl

Preparation time: 10 minutes

Cooking time: 10 minutes

Servings: 2

Ingredients:

Egg: 2

Cheddar cheese: 1 cup (shredded)

Mint: ¼ cup chopped

Onion: ½ cup chopped

Cucumber: ½ cup chopped

Tomato: ½ cup chopped

Lettuce: ½ cup chopped

Cabbage: ½ cup chopped

Salt: 1/2 tsp

Black pepper: ¼ tsp Fresh

coriander: ½ cup chopped

Directions:

Preheat a mini waffle maker if needed and grease it In a mixing bowl, beat eggs and add mint and shredded cheddar cheese to them Mix them all well and pour the mixture to the lower plate of the waffle maker Cook for at least 4 minutes to get the desired crunch

Remove from the heat and divide into four pieces when cool down Mix all the vegetable and seasoning and add chaffles too and serve Nutrition: 258 calories

20.6g fat 6.2g carbs

46.1g protein 2.1g sugars

1.7g fiber

320)Almond spinach chaffles

Preparation time: 15 minutes

Cooking time: 10 minutes

Servings: 2

Ingredients:

Cheddar cheese: 1/3 cup

Egg: 1

Spinach: 1/3 cup finely chopped

Lemon juice: 2 tbsp

Almond flour: 2 tbsp Baking

powder: 1/4 teaspoon ground

almonds: 2 tbsp Mozzarella

cheese: 1/3 cup Directions:

Mix cheddar cheese, egg, lemon juice, spinach, almond flour, almond ground, and baking powder together in a bowl

Preheat your waffle iron and grease it

In your mini waffle iron, shred half of the mozzarella cheese

Add the mixture to your mini waffle iron Again, shred the remaining mozzarella cheese on the mixture

Cook till the desired crisp is achieved

Make as many chaffles as your mixture and waffle maker allow
Nutrition: 258 calories

20.6g fat

6.2g carbs

46.1g protein

2.1g sugars

1.7g fiber

321) Pickled broccoli chaffles

Preparation time: 15 minutes

Cooking time: 10 minutes

Servings: 2

Ingredients:

Egg: 1

Boiled broccoli: ½ cup mashed

Cheddar cheese: ½ cup (shredded)

Pork panko: ½ cup

Pickle slices: 6-8 thin

Directions:

Mix egg, broccoli, cheese, and pork panko well together Pour a thin layer on a preheated waffle iron

Remove any excess juice from pickles Add pickle slices and pour again more mixture over the top

Cook the chaffle for around 5 minutes
Make as many chaffles as your mixture and waffle maker allow
Nutrition: 258 calories

20.6g fat

6.2g carbs

46.1g protein

2.1g sugars

1.7g fiber

322) Spiced mozzarella radish chaffles

Preparation time: 5 minutes

Cooking time: 10 minutes

Servings: 2

Ingredients: Egg: 1

Mozzarella cheese: ½ cup (shredded)

Thyme: 1 tsp

Radish: ½ cup finely grated

Allspice: a pinch

Salt and pepper: as per your taste

Coriander: ½ cup chopped

Directions:

Mix all the ingredients well together

Pour a layer on a preheated waffle iron

Cook the chaffle for around 5 minutes Make as many chaffles as

your mixture and waffle maker allow

Nutrition: 258 calories

20.6g fat 6.2g carbs

46.1g protein 2.1g sugars

1.7g fiber

323) Okra cauli chaffle

Preparation time: 10 minutes

Cooking time: 10 minutes

Servings: 2

Ingredients:

Cauliflower: 1/2 cup

Okra: ½ cup

Egg: 2

Mozzarella cheese: 1 cup (shredded)

Butter: 1 tbsp

Almond flour: 2 tbsp

Turmeric: ¼ tsp

Baking powder: ¼ tsp

Onion powder: a pinch

Garlic powder: a pinch

Salt: a pinch Directions:

In a deep saucepan, boil okra and cauliflower for five minutes or till it tenders, strain and set aside Mix all the remaining ingredients well together

Pour a thin layer on a preheated waffle iron

Remove any excess water from the vegetables and add a layer on the mixture

again, add more mixture over the top Cook the chaffle for around 5 minutes

Serve hot with your favorite keto sauce

Nutrition: 258 calories

20.6g fat

6.2g carbs

46.1g protein

2.1g sugars

1.7g fiber

324) Oniony pickled chaffles

Preparation time: 15 minutes

Cooking time: 10 minutes

Servings: 2

Ingredients:

Egg: 1

Onion: ½ cup finely chopped

Cheddar cheese: ½ cup (shredded) Pork panko: ½ cup

Pickle slices: 6-8 thin

Pickle juice: 1 tbsp Directions:

Mix egg, onion, cheese, and pork panko well together

Pour a thin layer on a preheated waffle iron Remove any excess juice from pickles Add pickle slices and pour again more mixture over the top

Cook the chaffle for around 5 minutes Make as many chaffles as your mixture and waffle maker allow Nutrition: 258 calories

20.6g fat

6.2g carbs

46.1g protein

2.1g sugars

1.7g fiber

Nutrition: 258 calories

20.6g fat

6.2g carbs

325) Flavored spinach chaffles

46.1g protein

Preparation time: 5 minutes

2.1g sugars

Cooking time: 10 minutes

1.7g fiber

Servings: 2

Ingredients:

Egg: 1

Cheddar cheese: ½ cup (shredded)

326) Veggies and olives chaffles salad

Thyme: 1 tsp

Preparation time: 10 minutes

Spinach: ½ cup chopped

Cooking time: 10 minutes

Allspice: a pinch

Servings: 2

Salt and pepper: as per your taste

Ingredients:

Coriander: ½ cup chopped

Egg: 2

Directions:

Cheddar cheese: 1 cup (shredded)

Mix all the ingredients well together

Onion: ½ cup thickly sliced

Pour a layer on a preheated waffle iron

Zucchini: ½ cup thickly sliced

Cook the chaffle for around 5 minutes

Cauliflower: 1 cup florets removed

Salt: 1/2 tsp

Make as many chaffles as your mixture and waffle maker allow

Black pepper: ¼ tsp

Butter: 1 tsp

Olives: ½ cup sliced   Fresh coriander: ½ cup chopped

Directions:

Preheat the oven

Add all the vegetables on the baking tray and sprinkle salt and pepper

Brush with oil and roast for 15 min

Preheat a mini waffle maker if needed and grease it

In a mixing bowl, beat eggs and add shredded cheddar cheese to them

Mix them all well and pour the mixture to the lower plate of the waffle maker   Cook for at least 4 minutes to get the desired crunch

Remove from the heat and divide into four pieces when cool down

Mix all the vegetable, olives, coriander, and chaffles together and serve Nutrition: 258 calories

20.6g fat

6.2g carbs

46.1g protein

2.1g sugars

1.7g fiber

327) Cauli spinach onion blend chaffles

Preparation time: 5 minutes

Cooking time: 10 minutes

Servings: 2

Ingredients:

Eggs: 2

Mozzarella: 1 cup shredded

Cream cheese: 2 tbsp

Butter: 1 tbsp

Onion: ½ cup

Tomato: ½ cup

Garlic powder: 1 tbsp

Pepper: ¼ tsp

Basil: ½ tsp

Spinach: ½ cup

Cauliflower florets: 1 cup

Salt: ¼ tsp

Directions:

Take a pan, heat butter and add onion and sauté for a minute Add tomatoes, spinach, and cauliflower and cook for 10 minutes

Preheat your mini waffle iron if needed

Mix all the above-mentioned ingredients in a bowl with cauliflower and blend using a hand blender Grease your waffle iron lightly

Cook your mixture in the mini waffle iron for at least 4 minutes

Serve hot with your favorite sauce

Make as many chaffles as your mixture and waffle maker allow

Nutrition: 258 calories

20.6g fat

6.2g carbs

46.1g protein

2.1g sugars

1.7g fiber

328) Plain spinach jalapeno chaffle

Preparation time: 4 minutes

Cooking time: 10 minutes

Servings: 2

Ingredients:

Egg: 2

Cheddar cheese: 1½ cup

Deli jalapeno: 16 slices Spinach: 1

cup chopped Directions:

Boil water and add spinach and boil for 5 minutes

Strain and drain to remove excess water

Preheat a mini waffle maker if needed In a mixing bowl, beat eggs and add half cheddar cheese to them and mix well Shred some of the remaining cheddar cheese to the lower plate of the waffle maker

Now pour the mixture to the shredded cheese and add in one spoon of spinach and spread

Add the cheese again on the top with around 4 slices of jalapeno and close the lid

Cook for at least 4 minutes to get the desired crunch and serve hot Make as many chaffles as your mixture allows

Nutrition: 258 calories

20.6g fat

6.2g carbs

46.1g protein

2.1g sugars

1.7g fiber

Ingredients:

Egg: 1

Mozzarella cheese: ½ cup (shredded)

Garlic cloves: 2 chopped

Pepper: ½ cup finely chopped

Onion: ½ cup finely chopped   Salt and pepper: as per your taste

Directions:

Mix all the ingredients well together

Pour a layer on a preheated waffle iron

Cook the chaffle for around 5 minutes

Make as many chaffles as your mixture and waffle maker allow Nutrition: 258 calories

20.6g fat 6.2g carbs 46.1g protein

2.1g sugars 1.7g fiber

Dessert & Cakes

329) Quick   onion peppery chaffles

Preparation time: 5 minutes
Cooking time: 10 minutes
Servings: 2

330) Flavorful crab cake

Preparation time: 10 minutes

Cooking time: 10 minutes

Servings: 4

Ingredients:

Oz lump crab meat

1 tsp old bay seasoning

½ tbsp dijon mustard

2 tbsp breadcrumbs

1 ½ tbsp mayonnaise

2 tbsp green onion, chopped

¼ cup bell pepper, chopped
Directions:

Add all ingredients into the mixing bowl and mix until well combined.

Make four even shape patties of bowl mixture and place on an instant vortex air fryer tray.

Lightly spray patties with a cooking spray.

Air fry at 370 f for 10 minutes.

Serve and enjoy.

Nutrition:

Calories 81
Fat 6.7 g
Carbohydrates 5.5 g
Sugar 1 g

Protein 9 g
Cholesterol 33 mg

331) Easy air fryer scallops

Preparation time: 10 minutes

Cooking time: 4 minutes

Servings: 2

Ingredients:

Scallops
Pepper
Salt
Directions:

Arrange scallops on instant vortex air fryer tray.

Spray scallops with cooking spray and season with pepper and salt.

Air fry scallops at 390 f for 2 minutes.

Turn scallops to the other side and air fry for 2 minutes more.

Serve and enjoy.

Nutrition:

Calories 106

Fat 0.9 g

Carbohydrates 2.9 g

Sugar 0 g

Protein 20.2 g

Cholesterol 40 mg

332) Delicious tilapia

Preparation time: 10 minutes

Cooking time: 8 minutes

Servings: 4

Ingredients:

4 tilapia fillets

¼ tsp cayenne pepper

½ tsp cumin

1 tsp garlic powder

1 tsp dried oregano

2 tsp brown sugar

1 ½ tbsp paprika

1 tsp salt

Directions:

In a small bowl, mix together paprika, cayenne pepper, cumin, garlic powder, oregano, brown sugar, and

salt and rub onto the fish fillets.

Spray fish fillets with cooking spray.

Arrange fish fillets on instant vortex air fryer tray and air fry at 400 f for 4 minutes.

Turn fish fillets to the other side and air fry for 4 minutes more.

Serve and enjoy.

Nutrition:

Calories 158

Fat 2 g

Carbohydrates 3.8 g

Sugar 1.9 g

Protein 32.2 g

Cholesterol 83 mg

333) Crispy coconut shrimp

Preparation time: 10 minutes

Cooking time: 12 minutes

Servings: 4

Ingredients:

1 lb. Shrimp, peeled and deveined

½ cup shredded coconut

1 cup breadcrumbs

2 egg whites, lightly beaten

½ cup flour

Pepper

Salt

Directions:

In a shallow dish, mix together flour, pepper, and salt.

In a second shallow dish add egg whites.

In a third shallow dish, mix together breadcrumbs, shredded coconut, and salt.

Coat shrimp with flour mixture then coat with egg mixture and finally coat with breadcrumb mixture.

Arrange shrimp on instant vortex air fryer tray.

Air fry at 400 f for 6 minutes.

Turn shrimp to the other side and air fry for 6 minutes more.

Serve and enjoy.

Nutrition:

Calories 342

Fat 6.9 g

Carbohydrates 34.7 g

Sugar 2.5 g

Protein 33.2 g

Cholesterol 239 mg

334) Shrimp scampi

Preparation time: 10 minutes

Cooking time: 10 minutes

Servings: 4

Ingredients:

1 lb. Shrimp

1 cup breadcrumbs

¼ tsp onion powder

¼ tsp paprika

¼ tsp cayenne pepper

¼ cup white wine

3 garlic cloves, minced

8 tbsp butter

½ tsp salt

Directions:

In a bowl, mix together breadcrumbs, onion powder, paprika, cayenne pepper, and salt. Set aside.

Melt butter in a pan over medium heat.

Add white wine and garlic in melted butter and stir well.

Remove pan from heat. Add breadcrumbs and shrimp in melted butter mixture and stir everything well and transfer to a baking dish.

Air fry at 350 f for 10 minutes.

Serve and enjoy.

Nutrition:

Calories 462

Fat 26.4 g

Carbohydrates 22.6 g

Sugar 1.9 g

Protein 29.9 g

Cholesterol 300 mg

335) Lemon pepper shrimp

Preparation time: 10 minutes

Cooking time: 8 minutes

Servings: 2

Ingredients:

Oz shrimp, peeled and deveined

¼ tsp garlic powder

¼ tsp paprika

1 tsp lemon pepper

1 fresh lemon juice

½ tbsp olive oil Directions:

In a mixing bowl, mix together garlic powder, paprika, lemon pepper, lemon juice, and olive oil.

Add shrimp and toss until shrimp is well coated.

Transfer shrimp on instant vortex air fryer tray and air fry at 400 f for 6-8 minutes or until firm.

Serve and enjoy.

Nutrition:

Calories 242

Fat 6.6 g

Carbohydrates 4.1 g

Sugar 0.6 g

Protein 39.1 g

Cholesterol 358 mg

336) Dijon garlic salmon

Preparation time: 10 minutes

Cooking time: 15 minutes

Servings: 4

Ingredients:

1 ½ lb. Salmon fillets

½ tbsp dijon mustard

1 tbsp garlic, minced

2 tbsp fresh lemon juice

2 tbsp olive oil

2 tbsp fresh parsley, chopped

1/8 tsp pepper

½ tsp salt

Directions:

Preheat the instant vortex air fryer to 400 f.

In a small bowl, mix together dijon mustard, garlic, lemon juice, olive oil, parsley, pepper, and salt.

Arrange salmon fillets on instant vortex air fryer oven tray.

Spread marinade over salmon fillets.

Bake salmon for 12-15 minutes.

Serve and enjoy.

Nutrition:

Calories 292

Fat 17.7 g

Carbohydrates 1.1 g

Sugar 0.2 g

Protein 33.4 g

Cholesterol 75 mg

337) Cajun shrimp

Preparation time: 10 minutes

Cooking time: 15 minutes

Servings: 4

Ingredients:

1 lb. Shrimp

2 tbsp parmesan cheese, grated

1 tsp garlic, minced

½ cup breadcrumbs

1 tsp olive oil

1 tbsp cajun seasoning Directions:

In a mixing bowl, mix together parmesan cheese, garlic, breadcrumbs, olive oil, and cajun seasoning.

Add shrimp and toss until well coated.

Arrange shrimp on instant vortex air fryer oven tray and air fry at 390 f for 5 minutes.

Serve and enjoy.

Nutrition:

Calories 209

Fat 4.4 g

Carbohydrates 11.7 g

Sugar 0.9 g

Protein 28.5 g

Cholesterol 241 mg

338) Cake with cream and strawberries

Preparation time: 10 minutes

cooking time: 15 minutes

servings: 2

Ingredients:

1 pure butter puff pastry to stretch

500g strawberries (clean and without skin)

1 bowl of custard

3 tbsp icing sugar baked at 210°c in the air fryer

Direction:

Unroll the puff pastry and place it on the baking sheet. Prick the bottom with a fork and spread the custard. Arrange the strawberries in a circle and sprinkle with icing sugar.

Cook in a fryer setting a 210°c for 15 minutes.

Remove the cake from the fryer with the tongs and let cool.

When serving sprinkle with icing sugar And why not, add some whipped cream.

Nutrition:

Calories 212.6

Fat 8.3 g

Carbohydrate 31.9 g

Sugars 17.4 g

Protein2.3 g

Cholesterol 21.4 mg

339) Caramelized pineapple and vanilla ice cream

Preparation time: 0-10 minutes cooking time: 15-30 minutes

servings: 4   people

Ingredients:

4 slices pineapple

20g butter

50g cane sugar Ice

cream/vanilla

cream

Direction:

Heat the air fryer at 1500c for 5 minutes. Let it brown for 15-30 minutes. Then, take it out and top with the cream.

Nutrition:

Calories 648

Fat 36.4g

Carbohydrates 73.2g

Sugar 61.6g

Protein 9.5g

Cholesterol 94mg

340) Apple pie

Preparation time: 20-30 minutes cooking time: 45-60 minutes

servings: 3

Ingredients:

600g flour

350g margarine

150g sugar

2 eggs

50g breadcrumbs

3 apples

75g raisins

75g sugar

1tsp cinnamon

Direction:

Put the flour, sugar, eggs, and margarine nuts in the blender just outside the refrigerator.

Mix everything until you get a compact and quite flexible mixture. Let it rest in the refrigerator for at least 30 minutes.

Preheat the air fryer at 1500c for 5 minutes.

Spread 2/3 of the mass of broken dough in 3-4 mm thick covering the previously floured and floured tank and making the edges adhere well, which should be at least 2 cm.

Place the breadcrumbs, apple slices, sugar, raisins, and cinnamon in the bottom
cover everything with the remaining dough and make holes in the top to allow steam to escape.

Cook for 40 minutes and then turn off the lower resistance.

Cook for another 20 minutes only with the upper resistance on. Once it has cooled, put it on a plate and serve.

Nutrition:

Calories 411

Fat 19.38g

Total carbohydrate 57.5g

Sugars 50g

Protein3.72g

Cholesterol0mg

341) Apple rotation

Preparation time: 10 – 20 minutes

Cooking time: 15 – 30 minutes
 servings: 6

Ingredients:

1 roll of rectangular puff pastry

220g of apples

50g of sugar

100g raisins

50g pine nuts

To taste breadcrumbs   Cinnamon powder to taste

Direction:

Put the raisins in warm water for at least 30 min. Meanwhile, peel the apples, remove the kernel, and cut them into thin slices. Pour the apples into a large bowl and add the dried raisins.

Add the cinnamon, sugar, and pine nuts, gently mix the ingredients and let stand.

Meanwhile, spread the puff pastry on a work surface with parchment paper. Sprinkle with the breadcrumbs, leaving a 2-3 cm border around. Place the mixture in the center of the dough and close the coating along.

Be careful not to tear the dough, close the sides tightly so that the contents do not come out during cooking.

Place the liner on the air fryer and cook over low temperature for about 25 min. When finished cooking, sprinkle the strudel with icing sugar and serve warm sliced.

Nutrition:

Calories 411

Fat 19.38g

Total carbohydrate 57.5g

Sugars 50g

Protein3.72g

Cholesterol0mg

342) Stuffed brioche crown

Preparation time: more than 30 minutes cooking time: 30 – 45 minutes
 servings: 8

Ingredients:

250g manitoba flour

250g flour 00

200 ml of warm milk

100 ml of warm water

50 ml of olive oil

25g baker's yeast

1 tbsp sugar

1 tsp fine salt

250g cooked ham

8 slices of emmental

Poppy seeds

1 tbsp of water

1 tsp olive oil

Direction:

Prepare the brioche crown and let it grow in a lightly floured and closed container with food wrap for about an hour.

Once the survey is finished, spread the dough with a rolling pin, forming a narrow rectangle. First place the ham and then the cheese, leaving about 2 cm of free edge around.

Roll everything up to get a cylinder. Cut approximately 2 cm slices and place them in the basket covered with baking paper by placing them side by side to form a crown.

Let the preparation rise for another hour before cooking. In the end, brush with a mixture of warm water and oil over the entire surface of the crown and sprinkle with poppy seeds.

Preheat the air fryer at 1800c for 5 minutes. Cook for 40 minutes.

Nutrition:

Calories 516

Fat 32g

Carbohydrates 39g

Sugars 7g

Protein 17g

Cholesterol 0mg

343) Fried cream

Preparation time: 10-20 minutes cooking time: 15-30 minutes
 servings: 8 Ingredients:

For the cream:

500 ml of whole milk

3 egg yolks

150 g of sugar

50 g flour

1 envelope vanilla sugar

Ingredients for the pie:

2 eggs

Unlimited breadcrumbs

1 tsp oil

Direction:

First prepare the custard once cooked, pour the cream into a dish previously covered with a transparent film and level well. Let cool at room temperature for about 2 hours.

Grease the basket and distribute it all over.

When the cream is cold, place it on a cutting board and cut it into dice pass each piece of cream first in the breadcrumbs, covering the 4 sides well in the beaten egg and then in the pie.

Place each part inside the basket. Set the temperature to 1500c.

Cook for 10 to 12 minutes, turning the pieces after 6 to 8 minutes.

The doses of this cream are enough to make 2 or even 3 kitchens in a row.

Nutrition:

Calories 355

Fat 18.37g

Carbohydrates 44.94g

Sugars 30.36g

Protein 4.81g

Cholesterol 45mg

344) Apple, cream, and hazelnut crumble

Preparation time: 10-20 minutes
cooking time: 15-30 minutes servings: 6

Ingredients:

4 golden apples

100 ml of water

50g cane sugar

50g of sugar

½ tbsp cinnamon

200 ml of fresh cream Chopped hazelnuts to taste

Direction:

In a bowl, combine the peeled apples, cut into small cubes, cane sugar, sugar, and cinnamon.

Pour the apples inside the basket, add the water. Set the air fryer to 1800c and simmer for 15 minutes depending on the type of apple used and the size of the pieces.

At the end, divide the apples in the serving glasses, cover with previously whipped   cream and sprinkle with chopped hazelnuts.

Nutrition:

Calories 828.8

Fat 44.8 g

Carbohydrate 120.6 g

Sugars54.2 g

Protein4.4 g

Cholesterol 29.5 mg

345) Fregolotta (venetian puff pastry pie) with hazelnuts

Preparation time: 10-20 minutes cooking time: 15-30 minutes

Servings: 8

Ingredients:

200g of flour

150g of sugar

100 g melted butter

100g hazelnuts

1 egg ½ sachet of yeast

Direction:

Do not finely chop the hazelnuts. In a large bowl, pour all the ingredients (the butter once melted should be cooled before using), mix lightly, without the dough becoming too liquid.

Place parchment paper on the bottom of the basket and pour the mixture into it. Spread it evenly.

Set the air fryer to 1800c and simmer for 15 minutes and then turn the cake.

Cook for an additional 5 minutes.

Let cool and sprinkle the cake with icing sugar.

Nutrition:

Calories 465

Carbohydrates 37g

Fat 25g

Sugars 3g

Protein 20g

Cholesterol 0mg

346) Frozen treats

Preparation time: 15-30 minutes

Cooking time: 15-30 minutes

servings: 8

Ingredient

s: 14

frozen

pieces Direction:

Place the handles, placing them on the parchment paper and place them on the basket.

Set the temperature to 1500c.

Cook everything for 25 min.

Nutrition:

Calories 111

Fat 20 g

Carbohydrates 21 g

Sugars 45g

Protein 7g

Cholesterol 0mg

347) Roscon of reyes (spanish king's cake)

Preparation time: 10-20 minutes

cooking time: 30-45 minutes

servings: 4

Ingredients:

2 puff pastries

100g almond flour

1 egg

75g of sugar

50g butter

1 vial of almond aroma

1 porcelain bean

Direction:

First, prepare the filling:

In a bowl mix the flour, egg, sugar, butter at room temperature and almond extract.

Stretch a puff pastry with the baking paper inside the basket. Prick with a fork and spread the filling well.

Place the bean inside, choosing an external position for the cake.

Cover with the second roll of puff pastry and weld the edges well. Brush the surface with an egg yolk diluted with milk and decorate with small incisions.

Set the temperature to 1800c. Bake the pie for 25 minutes

Turn the baking paper half a turn and cook for another 10 minutes.

Tradition says that the person who finds the hidden bean becomes the "king" of the day.

Nutrition:

Calories 1426

Fat 10.54g

Carbohydrates 56.54g

Sugar 23.51g

Protein 6.58g

Cholesterol 29mg

348) Nut cake

Preparation time: 10-20 minutes

cooking time: 30-45 minutes servings: 10 Ingredients:

250 g of walnuts

150g maïzena

4 medium eggs

200g of butter (room temperature)

1 sachet of yeast

1 sachet of vanilla sugar

200g of sugar

Direction:

Chop the nuts with 50 g of sugar. Using a food processor, beat the butter with the remaining sugar until you get a shiny and foamy mixture.

Add the eggs one by one, making sure the mixture is still soft, then add the vanilla.

Add the chopped nuts with the sugar and then the cornstarch that will sift with the yeast.

Butter and flour the basket, then pour the mixture in the center.

Set the air fryer at 1800c.

Cook for 45 minutes (turn off the lower heating element 40 minutes later). Let cool before serving.

Nutrition: Calories 440 Fat 20.48g

Carbohydrate 62.22g Sugars 49.65g

Protein 3.72g Cholesterol 53mg

349) Italian cake

Preparation time: 10-20 minutes cooking time: 30-45 minutes

 servings: 8

Ingredients:

250g of potato starch

150g of flour 00 (flour 55)

250g of sugar

6 eggs

50 g butter

1 sachet of yeast

Powdered sugar

Direction:

Melt the butter in a small saucepan and let it cool.

Beat the eggs with the fine sugar until you get a light and frothy mixture. Add the flour, starch, sifted yeast, melted butter and mix until a homogeneous mixture is obtained.

Butter and flour the basket and pour the preparation into it.

Set the temperature to 1800c and cook the cake for 35 min.

Remove the cake from the bowl, let it cool and sprinkle with icing sugar.

Nutrition:

Calories 440

Carbohydrates 40g

Fat 30g

Sugars 28g

Protein 4g

Cholesterol 65mg

350) Marble cake

Preparation time: 10-20 minutes
cooking time: 45-60 minutes
servings: 10

Ingredients:

190g butter

1g bag of vanilla sugar

12g baking powder

375g flour

22g cocoa powder

4g medium eggs

225g of sugar

165 ml of milk

Salt (a pinch)

Direction:

Put the previously softened butter into small pieces in a bowl with the sugar, mount the ingredients until a white and foamy cream forms.

Add the eggs at room temperature, one by one, the salt and beat about 5 minutes until you get a mixture without lumps. Add the flour (except 30 g that will keep aside), the yeast and vanilla sugar sifted alternately with the milk.

Mix the ingredients well, then divide them evenly and add the remaining flour in a bowl and the sifted cocoa in another.

Butter and flour the basket and first place the transparent mixture divided into three separate parts. Do the same with the dark mixture by filling the remaining gaps between the light mixture.

To get the veined effect, rotate a fork from top to bottom through the two colors of the mixture.

Set the air fryer to 1800c and cook for 40 minutes and then turn off the lower resistance.

Cook for another 10 min. Control the baking of the cake with the tip of a knife.

Nutrition:

Calories 195

Fat 7.6g

Carbohydrates 28g

Sugars 14g

Protein 3.5g

Cholesterol 47mg

351) Genoves cake

Preparation time: 10-20 minutes cooking time: 30-45 minutes

servings: 10 Ingredients:

6 eggs

190g of sugar

150g of flour 00 (flour 55)

75g potato starch

2g vanilla sugar

Direction:

In a bowl, beat the eggs with the sugar until you get a light and smooth mixture. Add the sifted flour, starch and vanilla sugar and mix with a whisk until a homogeneous mixture is obtained.

Butter and flour the basket, then pour the mixture.

Set the air fryer to 1800c and simmer for 35 minutes. Nutrition:

Calories 74

Fat1.83g

Carbohydrate10.91g

Sugars 5.08g

Protein 3.83g

Cholesterol 74mg

352) Frozen sorrentino gnocchi

Preparation time: 15-30 minutes

Cooking time: 0 – 15 minutes

servings: 2

Ingredients: 550 g

sorrentino gnocchi

Direction:

Pour the gnocchi in the basket and cook for 13 minutes at 1500c mixing once halfway through cooking.

Nutrition:

Calories 170

Carbohydrates 30g

Fat 2g

Sugars 11g

Protein 6g

Cholesterol 5mg

353) Khachapuri (georgian bread)

Preparation time: more than 30 minutes

cooking time: 15 – 30 minutes

servings: 4

Ingredients:

500g of flour

450g whole yogurt

½ tsp baking soda

½ tsp salt

150 g ricotta

100g provokes smoked

150g greek feta cheese

4 tbsp fine parsley

Direction:

Prepare the khachapuri dough by mixing all the ingredients until a smooth and homogeneous mixture is obtained. Divide the dough into 8 equal parts.

Form 8 balls cover them with a clean cloth. Let them rest in a warm place and away from drafts. After about 1 hour of lifting, start spreading the dough.

Meanwhile, prepare the filling by grating provokes smoked and the feta cheese and then mix with the ricotta and parsley.

Spread the 8 balls by hand in circles of 10 to 15 cm, fill 4 circles with the previously prepared filling and close with the other 4. Now roll the 4 khachapuri with a roller until you get a diameter of the size of the basket.

Grease the bottom of the basket and place 1 khachapuri. Also grease the surface and prick with a fork.

Set the air fryer to 1800c and cook each khachapuri for 15 minutes.

Nutrition:

Calories 556

Fat 33g

Carbohydrates 37g

Sugars 3.6g

Protein 28g

Cholesterol 181mg

354) Sweet and sour onions

Preparation time: 10-20 minutes

Cooking time: 30-45 minutes servings: 8

Ingredients:

600g of borretano onions

30g butter

30g of sugar

50g of modena balsamic vinegar

Direction:

First peel and wash the onions.

Add the butter and set the air fryer to 1600c

Melt the butter for 2 minutes.

Add the sugar and vinegar and cook for another 3 minutes.

Then pour the onions and cook them for 30 minutes or to the desired cooking point (this may vary depending on the size of the onions).

They can be served as an appetizer or to accompany meat dishes.

Nutrition:

Calories 80

Carbohydrates 17g

Fat 1g

Sugars 12g

Protein 1g

Cholesterol 0mg

355) Frozen paella

Preparation time: 15-30 minutes

Cooking time: 15-30 minutes

servings: 2

Ingredients:

600 g of paella

Direction:

Pour the paella in the basket and set the temperature to 1500c.

Cook for 15 minutes, mixing once in the middle of cooking.

Nutrition:

Calories 315

Carbohydrates 0g

Fat 9g

Protein 0g

Sugar 0g

Cholesterol 0mg

356) Spice bread

Preparation time: 10 – 20 minutes cooking time: 0 – 15 minutes

 servings: 10

Ingredients:

Ingredients for 30 - 35 cookies:

350g flour

160g of sugar

150g of butter

1 egg

1 pinch of salt

150g of honey

2 tsp cinnamon

¼ tsp nutmeg

2 tsp ginger

½ tsp of clove (powder)

Direction:

Put all the ingredients in a blender (the butter should be cold as soon as it comes out of the fridge).

Mix everything until you get a compact and sufficiently elastic mixture. Let it rest in the refrigerator for about 2 hours.

Then spread a 4 mm thick puff pastry with the rolling pin. Use templates to cut the dough in several ways.

Bake the cookies for 7 minutes at 1800c, and then rotate the baking paper.

Cook for additional 5 minutes, after cooling. Decorate to your liking.

Nutrition:

calories

100 Fat 0g

Carbohydrates 21g

Sugar 6g

Protein 3g

Cholesterol 0mg

357) Grilled curried fruit

Preparation time: 10 minutes   cooking time: 5 minutes
serves 6 to 8

350°f grill

Fast, vegetarian, gluten-free

If you've never had grilled fruit before, here's a wonderful introduction. Grilling caramelizes the sugars in fruits, brings out their flavor, and even turns fruit that's not quite ripe into a sweet dessert. Serve with some sherbet or ice cream for a cooling contrast.

2 peaches

2 firm pears

2 plums

2 tablespoons melted butter

1 tablespoon honey

2 to 3 teaspoons curry powder

Cut the peaches in half, remove the pits, and cut each half in half again. Cut the pears in half, core them, and remove the stem. Cut each half in half again. Do the same with the plums.

Spread a large sheet of heavy-duty foil on your work surface. Arrange the fruit on the foil and drizzle with the butter and honey. Sprinkle with the curry powder.

Wrap the fruit in the foil, making sure to leave some air space in the packet.

Put the foil package in the basket and grill for 5 to 8 minutes, shaking the basket once during the cooking time, until the fruit is soft and tender.

Ingredient tip: cut pears oxidize quickly, resulting in brown fruit. You can prevent browning by squeezing a little bit of fresh lemon juice onto the slices. The ascorbic acid in the lemon works to combat oxidation.

Nutrition:

calories

100 Fat 0g

Carbohydrates 21g

Sugar 6g

Protein 3g

Cholesterol 0mg

358) Apple peach cranberry crisp

Preparation time: 10 minutes

Cooking time: 12 minutes

Serves 8

380°f bake

Family favorite, vegetarian

A crisp, or a crumble, is a combination of cooked fruit topped with a sweet streusel. This classic dessert is perfect for fall dinners. Serve with a scoop of ice cream or softly whipped cream flavored with vanilla.

1 apple, peeled and chopped

2 peaches, peeled and chopped

⅓ cup dried cranberries

2 tablespoons honey

⅓ cup brown sugar

¼ cup flour

½ cup oatmeal

3 tablespoons softened butter

In a 6-by-6-by-2-inch pan, combine the apple, peaches, cranberries, and honey, and mix well.

In a medium bowl, combine the brown sugar, flour, oatmeal, and butter, and mix until crumbly. Sprinkle this mixture over the fruit in the pan.

Bake for 10 to 12 minutes or until the fruit is bubbly and the topping is golden brown. Serve warm.

Substitution tip: other fruits can be used in this recipe. Try chopped plums or nectarines instead of the apple and peaches. Or use golden raisins or currants in   place of the   dried cranberries.

Nutrition:

calories

100 Fat 0g

Carbohydrates 21g

Sugar 6g

Protein 3g

Cholesterol 0mg

359) Orange cornmeal cake

Preparation time: 7 minutes cooking time: 23 minutes

 serves 8

340°f bake

Family favorite, vegetarian

Cornmeal adds wonderful flavor and a bit of crunch to this tender cake recipe. An orange glaze is poured over the cake when it's still hot and soaks into the crumb. Serve this cake with a cup of coffee for a breakfast treat or afternoon snack.

Nonstick baking spray with flour

1¼ cups all-purpose flour

⅓ cup yellow cornmeal

¾ cup white sugar

1 teaspoon baking soda

¼ cup safflower oil

1¼ cups orange juice, divided

1 teaspoon vanilla

¼ cup powdered sugar

Spray a 6-by-6-by-2-inch baking pan with nonstick spray and set aside.

In a medium bowl, combine the flour, cornmeal, sugar, baking soda, safflower oil, 1 cup of the orange juice, and vanilla, and mix well.

Pour the batter into the baking pan and place in the air fryer. Bake for 23 minutes or until a toothpick inserted in the center of the cake comes out clean.

Remove the cake from the basket and place on a cooling rack. Using a toothpick, make about 20 holes in the cake.

In a small bowl, combine remaining ¼ cup of orange juice and the powdered sugar and stir well. Drizzle this mixture over the hot cake slowly so the cake absorbs it.

Cool completely, then cut into wedges to serve.

Did you know? To test for doneness when baking cakes, there are a few rules. A cake should spring back lightly when gently touched with a finger. Or, you can insert a clean toothpick into the cake; it should come out clean. Finally, when a cake is done, it starts to pull away from the sides of the baking pan slightly.

Nutrition:

calories 253 Fat

0g

Carbohydrates 21g

Sugar 6g

Protein 3g

Cholesterol 0mg

360) Black forest hand pies

Preparation time: 10 minutes   cooking time: 15 minutes

 serves 6

300°f bake

Family favorite, vegetarian

Black forest torte is an old-world cake with chocolate and cherries. This easy recipe is fun to make, and kids especially love it. The chocolate and cherries are encased in puff pastry, which cooks to perfection in the air fryer. These tastes delicious warm or cold.

3 tablespoons milk or dark chocolate chips

2 tablespoons thick, hot fudge sauce

2 tablespoons chopped dried cherries

1 (10-by-15-inch) sheet puff pastry, thawed

1 egg white, beaten

2 tablespoons sugar

½ teaspoon cinnamon

In a small bowl, combine the chocolate chips, fudge sauce, and dried cherries.

Roll out the puff pastry on a floured surface. Cut into 6 squares with a sharp knife.

Divide the chocolate chip mixture onto the center of each puff pastry square. Fold the squares in half to make triangles. Firmly press the edges with the tines of a fork to seal.

Brush the triangles on all sides sparingly with the beaten egg white.

Sprinkle the tops with sugar and cinnamon.

Place in the air fryer basket and bake for 15 minutes or until the triangles are golden brown. The filling will be hot, so cool for at least 20 minutes before serving.

Air fryer tip: make sure that these little pies are not touching each other in the air fryer so they brown and crisp on all sides.

Nutrition:

calories 100 Fat

0g

Carbohydrates 21g

Sugar 6g

Protein 3g

Cholesterol 0mg

361) Marble cheesecake

Preparation time: 10 minutes   cooking time: 20 minutes

 serves 8

320°f bake

Family favorite, vegetarian

A cheesecake cooked in the air fryer seems improbable, but it works! This cheesecake is a combination of vanilla and chocolate. It's not only delicious, it's gorgeous, too. Splurge and enjoy for dessert after a weeknight meal.

1 cup graham cracker crumbs

3 tablespoons softened butter 1½ (8-ounce) packages cream cheese, softened

⅓ cup sugar

2 eggs, beaten

1 tablespoon

flour 1

teaspoon

vanilla

¼ cup chocolate syrup

For the crust, combine the graham cracker crumbs and butter in a small bowl and mix well. Press into the bottom of a 6-by-6-by-2-inch baking pan and put in the freezer to set.

For the filling, combine the cream cheese and sugar in a medium bowl and mix well. Beat in the eggs, one at a time. Add the flour and vanilla.

Remove ⅔ cup of the filling to a small bowl and stir in the chocolate syrup until combined.

Pour the vanilla filling into the pan with the crust. Drop the chocolate filling over the vanilla filling by the spoonful. With a clean butter knife stir the fillings in a zigzag pattern to marbleize them.

Bake for 20 minutes or until the cheesecake is just set.

Cool on a wire rack for 1 hour, then chill in the refrigerator until the cheesecake is firm.

Substitution tip: using this basic recipe, you can make other flavors. Add ½ cup chocolate syrup and don't divide the batter for a chocolate cheesecake. Omit the chocolate syrup and add about ⅓ cup of lemon curd for a lemon cheesecake.

Nutrition:

calories 311 Fat

0g

Carbohydrates 21g

Sugar 6g

Protein 3g

Cholesterol 0mg

362) Black and white brownies

Preparation time: 10 minutes
cooking time: 20 minutes
Servings: 1 dozen brownies

340°f bake

Family favorite, vegetarian

Who doesn't love brownies? In the air fryer, the brownies stay moist and deeply rich, but get the most wonderful crunchy and crisp top. This easy recipe should quickly become part of your regular air frying repertoire.

1 egg

¼ cup brown sugar

2 tablespoons white sugar

2 tablespoons safflower oil

1 teaspoon vanilla

¼ cup cocoa powder

⅓ cup all-purpose flour

¼ cup white chocolate chips

Nonstick baking spray with flour

In a medium bowl, beat the egg with the brown sugar and white sugar. Beat in the oil and vanilla.

Add the cocoa powder and flour and stir just until combined. Fold in the white chocolate chips.

Spray a 6-by-6-by-2-inch baking pan with nonstick spray. Spoon the brownie batter into the pan.

Bake for 20 minutes or until the brownies are set when lightly touched with a finger. Let cool for 30 minutes before slicing to serve.

Cooking tip: you measure cocoa powder just like you measure flour: spoon it lightly into a measuring cup and level off the top with the back of a knife. Never scoop flour or dry ingredients into a measuring cup because that adds too much to the recipe and your cookies, cakes, and bars will be dense and heavy.

Nutrition: calories 81

Fat 4

Carbohydrates 23 Sugar 5 Protein 2

Cholesterol 0mg

363) Chocolate peanut butter molten cupcakes

Preparation time: 10 minutes
cooking time: 10 to 13 minutes
Servings: 8 cupcakes

320°f bake

Family favorite, vegetarian

Molten cupcakes are cakes that are slightly under baked, so the center stays runny. This recipe is a bit different: a ball of peanut butter and powdered sugar is added to the middle of each cupcake before baking. It softens as the cake bakes, creating a molten middle of sweet peanut butter. Serve these cupcakes warm with vanilla ice cream.

Nonstick baking spray with flour

1⅓ cups chocolate cake mix (from 15ounce box) 1 egg

1 egg yolk

¼ cup safflower oil

¼ cup hot water

⅓ cup sour cream

3 tablespoons peanut butter

1 tablespoon powdered sugar

Double up 16 foil muffin cups to make 8 cups. Spray each lightly with nonstick spray; set aside.

In a medium bowl, combine the cake mix, egg, egg yolk, safflower oil, water, and sour cream, and beat until combined.

In a small bowl, combine the peanut butter and powdered sugar and mix well. Form this mixture into 8 balls.

Spoon about ¼ cup of the chocolate batter into each muffin cup and top with a peanut butter ball. Spoon remaining batter on top of the peanut butter balls to cover them.

Arrange the cups in the air fryer basket, leaving some space between each. Bake for 10 to 13 minutes or until the tops look dry and set.

Let the cupcakes cool for about 10 minutes, then serve warm.

Ingredient tip: save the rest of the chocolate cake mix in a sealed heavyduty plastic bag. Be sure to mark it with the date that you used it. Use it within two weeks—maybe to make more batches of this recipe!

Nutrition:

calories

100 Fat 0g

Carbohydrates 21g

Sugar 6g

Protein 3g

Cholesterol 0mg

364) Chocolate peanut butter bread pudding

Preparation time: 10 minutes cooking time: 10 to 12 minutes
 serves 8

330°f bake

Family favorite, vegetarian

Bread pudding is the ultimate comfort food. The addition of chocolate and peanut butter adds a subtle richness to this recipe and intensifies the flavors.

Serve with heavy whipped cream to double the indulgence.

Nonstick baking spray with flour

1 egg

1 egg yolk

¾ cup chocolate milk

2 tablespoons cocoa powder

3 tablespoons brown sugar

3 tablespoons peanut butter

1 teaspoon vanilla

5 slices firm white bread, cubed

Spray a 6-by-6-by-2-inch baking pan with nonstick spray.

In a medium bowl, combine the egg, egg yolk, chocolate milk, cocoa, brown sugar, peanut butter, and vanilla, and mix until combined. Stir in the bread cubes and let soak for 10 minutes.

Spoon this mixture into the prepared pan. Bake for 10 to 12 minutes or until the pudding is firm to the touch.

Substitution tip: use different types of bread in this recipe. You could use cubed doughnuts or try a quick bread such as banana bread or peanut butter bread.

Nutrition:

calories

102 Fat 0g

Carbohydrates 21g

Sugar 6g

Protein 3g

Cholesterol 0mg

365) Big chocolate chip cookie

Preparation time: 7 minutes cooking time: 9 minutes

 serves 4

300°f bake

Fast, family favorite, vegetarian

Everyone loves chocolate chip cookies. But have you ever made one that was 6 inches in diameter?

This fun recipe makes one big cookie that serves four people. Everyone breaks off a piece to enjoy.   This cookie   is especially wonderful served warm.

Nonstick baking spray with flour

3 tablespoons softened butter

⅓ cup plus 1 tablespoon brown sugar

1 egg yolk

½ cup flour

2 tablespoons ground white chocolate

¼ teaspoon baking soda

½ teaspoon vanilla

¾ cup chocolate chips

In medium bowl, beat the butter and brown sugar together until fluffy. Stir in the egg yolk.

Add the flour, white chocolate, baking soda, and vanilla, and mix well. Stir in the chocolate chips.

Line a 6-by-6-by-2-inch baking pan with parchment paper. Spray the parchment paper with nonstick baking spray with flour.

Spread the batter into the prepared pan, leaving a ½-inch border on all sides.

Bake for about 9 minutes or until the cookie is light brown and just barely set.

Remove the pan from the air fryer and let cool for 10 minutes. Remove the cookie from the pan, remove the parchment paper, and let cool on a wire rack.

Substitution tip: you can use other types of chocolate chips in this recipe. Try milk chocolate chips or butterscotch chips. Or add about ¼ cup chopped pecans or cashews when you stir in the chocolate chips.

Nutrition:

calories

309 Fat 0g

Carbohydrates 21g

Sugar 6g

Protein 3g

Cholesterol 0mg

366) Frosted peanut butter cookie

Preparation time: 10 minutes   cooking time: 10 minutes

serves 4

310°f bake

Family favorite, vegetarian

A giant peanut butter cookie topped with melted chocolate is the perfect dessert on a weeknight. Eat this cookie warm while the frosting is still soft for an indulgent treat.

3   tablespoons butter,   at room temperature

⅓ cup plus 1 tablespoon brown sugar

1 egg yolk

⅔ cup flour

5 tablespoons peanut butter, divided

¼ teaspoon baking soda

1 teaspoon vanilla

½ cup semisweet chocolate chips

In a medium bowl, beat the butter and brown sugar together until fluffy. Stir in the egg yolk.

Add the flour, 3 tablespoons of the peanut butter, the baking soda, and vanilla, and mix well.

Line a 6-by-6-by-2-inch baking pan with parchment paper.

Spread the batter into the prepared pan, leaving a ½-inch border on all sides.

Bake for 7 to 10 minutes or until the cookie is light brown and just barely set.

Remove the pan from the air fryer and let cool for 10 minutes. Remove the cookie from the pan, remove the parchment paper, and let cool on a wire rack.

In a small heatproof cup, combine the chocolate chips with the remaining 2 tablespoons of peanut butter. Bake for 1 to 2 minutes or until the chips are melted. Stir to combine and spread on the cookie.

Variation tip: you can double or triple this recipe. You can also serve the cookie unfrosted, or combine 2

tablespoons soft butter, 2 tablespoons peanut butter, and ½ cup powdered sugar, mix well, and use to frost the cookie.

Nutrition: calories 491

Fat 0g

Carbohydrates 21g Sugar 6g

Protein 3g Cholesterol 0mg

367) Chocolate mug cake

Preparation time: 7 minutes

Cooking time: 13 minutes serves 3

Ingredients:

½ cup of cocoa powder

½ cup stevia powder

1 cup coconut cream

1 package cream cheese, room temperature

1 tbsp. Vanilla extract

1 tbsp. Butter

Directions:

Preheat the smart air fryer oven for 5 minutes at 350°f.

In a mixing bowl, combine all the listed ingredients using a hand mixer until fluffy.

Pour into greased mugs.

Place the mugs in the fryer basket and bake for 13 minutes at 350°f.

Serve when cool.

Nutrition:

calories

100 Fat

0g

Carbohydrates 21g

Sugar 6g

Protein 3g

Cholesterol 0mg

368) Air fryer chocolate cake

Preparation time: 6

minutes cooking time: 35

minutes serves 9

Ingredients:

½cups hot water

1 tsp. Vanilla

¼cups olive oil

½cups almond milk

1 egg

½ tsp. Salt

¾ tsp. Baking soda

¾ tsp. Baking powder

½cups unsweetened cocoa powder

2cups almond flour

1 cup brown sugar

Directions:

Preheat your smart air fryer oven to 356 °f.

Stir all dry ingredients together and then stir in wet ingredients.

Add hot water last.

The batter should be thin.

Pour cake batter into a pan that fits into the fryer.

Bake for 35 minutes.

Nutrition:

calories 378

Fat9g

Carbs5g

Protein 4g

369) Air fried biscuit donuts

Preparation time: 7 minutes

cooking time: 5 minutes

Serves 8

Ingredients:

Pinch of allspice

4 tbsp. Dark brown sugar

1 tsp. Cinnamon

1/3cups granulated sweetener

3 tbsp. Melted coconut oil

1 can of biscuits

Directions:

Mix allspice, sugar, sweetener, and cinnamon.

Take out biscuits from can and with a circle cookie cutter, cut holes from centers, and place into the air fryer. Cook 5 minutes at 350 °f

As batches are cooked, use a brush to coat with melted coconut oil and dip each into sugar mixture.

Serve warm!

Nutrition: calories

378 Fat9g

Carbs5g

Protein 4g

370) Chocolate soufflé

Preparation time: 7 minutes

cooking time: 12 minutes serves 2

Ingredients:

2 tbsp. Almond flour

½ tsp. Vanilla

3 tbsp. Sweetener

2 separated eggs

¼cups melted coconut oil   3 oz.

Of semi-sweet chocolate, chopped

Directions:

Preheat the smart air fryer oven to 330
°f.

Brush coconut oil and sweetener onto ramekins.

Melt coconut oil and chocolate together.

Beat egg yolks well, adding vanilla and sweetener.

Stir in flour and ensure there are no lumps.

Whisk egg whites till they reach peak state and fold them into chocolate mixture.

Pour batter into ramekins and place into the smart air fryer oven, then cook for 12 minutes.

Serve with powdered sugar dusted on top.

Nutrition facts nutrition per serving:

Nutrition: calories

378 Fat9g

Carbs5g

Protein 4g

371) Saucy fried bananas

Preparation time: 7 minutes

cooking time: 10 minutes serves 2

Ingredients:

1 large egg

¼ cup cornstarch

¼ cup plain breadcrumbs

3 bananas, halved crosswise

Cooking oil

Chocolate sauce

Directions:

Preheat your smart air fryer oven to 350 °f.

In a small bowl, beat the egg.

In another bowl, place the cornstarch.

Place the breadcrumbs in a different bowl.

Dip the bananas in the cornstarch, then the egg, and then the breadcrumbs.

Spray the basket with cooking oil. Place the bananas in the basket and spray them with cooking oil.

Cook for 5 minutes.

Open the air fryer and flip the bananas then cook for an additional 2 minutes. Transfer the bananas to plates.

Drizzle the chocolate sauce over the bananas and serve.

Nutrition:

calories 378

Fat9g

Carbs5g

Protein 4g

372) Crusty apple hand pies

Preparation time: 7 minutes

Cooking time: 8 minutes serves 6

Ingredients:

15-oz. No-sugar-added apple pie filling

1 store-bought crust

Directions:

Lay out pie crust and slice into equalsized squares.

Place 2 tbsp. Filling into each square and seal crust with a fork

Pour into the oven rack/basket.

Place the rack on the middle-shelf of the smart air fryer oven.

Set temperature to 390°f and set time to 8 minutes until golden in color.

Nutrition: calories

378 Fat9g

Carbs5g Protein 4g

373) Blueberry lemon muffins

Preparation time: 7 minutes

Cooking time: 8 minutes

Serves 12

Ingredients:

1 tsp. Vanilla

Juice and zest of 1 lemon

2 eggs

1 cup blueberries

½cups cream

¼cups avocado oil

½ cup monk

fruit 2 ½cups

almond flour

Directions:

Mix monk fruit and flour.

In another bowl, mix vanilla, egg, lemon juice, and cream.

Add mixtures together and blend well.

Spoon batter into cupcake holders   Place in the smart air fryer oven, then bake for 8 minutes at 320 °f, checking at 6 minutes to ensure you don't over bake them.

Nutrition: calories

378 Fat9g

Carbs5g

Protein 4g

374) Cream cheese wontons

Preparation time: 5 minutes

Cooking time: 5 minutes

Serves 16

Ingredients:

1 egg mixed with a bit of water

Wonton wrappers

½cup powdered erythritol   8 oz.

Softened cream cheese olive oil

Directions:

Mix   sweetener   and   cream cheese together.

Lay out four wontons at a time and cover with a dish towel to prevent drying out.

Place ½ of a tsp. Of cream cheese mixture into each wrapper

Dip finger into egg/water mixture and fold diagonally to form a triangle.

Seal edges well and repeat the same with the remaining ingredients.

Place filled wontons into the smart air fryer oven and cook 5 minutes at 400 °f, shaking halfway through cooking.

Nutrition:

calories 378

Fat9g

Carbs5g

Protein 4g

375) Air fryer cinnamon rolls

Preparation time: 2 hours 11 minutes

Cooking time: 5 minutes

Serves 8

Ingredients:

1 ½ tbsp. Cinnamon

¾cups brown sugar

¼cups melted coconut oil   1 lb.

Frozen bread dough, thawed

Glaze:

½ tsp. Vanilla

1 ¼cups powdered erythritol

2tbsp. Softened ghee 3 oz. Softened

  cream cheese

Directions:

Lay out bread dough and roll out into a rectangle.

Brush melted ghee over the dough and leave a 1-inch border along edges.

Mix cinnamon and sweetener and then sprinkle over dough.

Roll dough tightly and slice into 8 pieces.

Let sit for 2 hours to rise

To make the glaze, simply mix the glaze ingredients till smooth.

Once rolls rise, place into the air fryer and cook 5 minutes at 350 °f.

Serve rolls drizzled in cream cheese glaze.

Enjoy!

Nutrition:

calories 378

Fat9g

Carbs5g

Protein 4g

376) Cherry-choco bars

Preparation time: 7 minutes

Cooking time: 15 minutes

Serves 8

Ingredients:

¼ tsp. Salt

½ cup almonds, sliced

½ cup chia seeds

½ cup dark chocolate, chopped

½ cup dried cherries, chopped

½ cup prunes, pureed

½ cup quinoa, cooked

¾ cup almond butter

1/3 cup honey

2 cups oats

2 tbsp. Coconut oil

Directions:

Preheat the smart air fryer oven to 375°f.

In a bowl, combine the oats, quinoa, chia seeds, almond, cherries, and chocolate.

In a saucepan, heat the almond butter, honey, and coconut oil.

Pour the butter mixture over the dry mix, then add salt and prunes and mix until well combined.

Pour over a baking dish that can fit inside the air fryer.

Bake for 15 minutes.

Let it cool before slicing into bars.

Nutrition:

calories 378 Fat9g

Carbs5g

Protein 4g

377) Cinnamon fried bananas

Preparation time: 7 minutes

Cooking time: 10 minutes

Serves 3

Ingredients:

1 cup panko breadcrumbs

3 tbsp. Cinnamon

½ cups almond flour

3 egg whites

8 ripe bananas

3 tbsp. Coconut oil   Directions:

Heat coconut oil and add breadcrumbs, then mix around 3 minutes until golden and pour into a bowl.

Peel and cut bananas in half.

Roll the half of each banana into flour, eggs, and crumb mixture.

Place into the smart air fryer oven. Cook 10 minutes at 280 °f.

Enjoy!

Nutrition: calories

221 Fat9g

Carbs5g

Protein 4g

378) Air fryer doughnuts

Preparation time: 35 mins

Cooking time: 60 minutes

Serves 8 (serving size: 1 doughnut)

Ingredients

1/4 cup warm water, warmed (100f to 110f)

One tablespoon active yeast

1/4 cup, plus half tsp. Granulated sugar, divided

2 cups (about 8 1/2 oz.) All-purpose flour

1/4 teaspoon kosher salt

1/4 cup whole milk, at room

temperature

Two tablespoons unsalted butter,

melted

One large egg, beaten

1 cup (about 4 oz.) Powdered sugar

Four teaspoons tap water

How to make it

Step 1

Mix together water, yeast, and 1/2 teaspoon of the granulated sugar in a small bowl; let stand until foamy, around five minutes. Combine flour, salt, and remaining 1/4 cup granulated sugar in a medium bowl. Add yeast mixture, milk, butter, and egg; stir it with a wooden spoon until a soft dough comes together. Turn dough out onto a lightly floured surface and knead until smooth, 1 to 2 minutes. Switch dough to a lightly greased tub. Cover and let rise in a warm place until doubled in volume, around 1 hour.

Step 2

Turn dough out onto a lightly floured surface. Gently roll to 1/4-inch thickness. Cut out eight doughnuts using a 3-inch round cutter and a 1-inch round cutter to delete core: place doughnuts and doughnuts holes on a lightly floured surface. Cover loosely with plastic wrap and let stand for about 30 minutes, until doubled in volume.

Step 3

Place two doughnuts and two doughnuts holes in a single layer in air fryer pan, and cook at 350 ° f until golden brown,

4 to 5 minutes. Continue with doughnuts and holes remaining on.

Step 4

Whisk powdered sugar together and tap water until smooth in a medium bowl. In a glaze, dip doughnuts and doughnut holes, place them on a wire rack set above a rimmed baking sheet to allow excess glaze to drip off. Let stand for about 10 minutes, until the glaze hardens.

Nutrition:

calories 378

Fat9g

Carbs5g

Protein 4g

379) Choc chip air fryer cookies

Preparation time: 10 minutes

Cooking time: 16 minutes

Servings: 3

Category: dessert

Ingredients

75 grams self raising flour

100 grams butter

75 grams brown sugar

75 grams milk chocolate

30 milliliters honey

30 milliliters whole milk

Directions:

Beat the butter until smooth and fluffy. Add the butter to the sugar and beat together in a smooth mixture. Now add and mix in the milk, sugar, chocolate (broken into small chunks/chips), and flour. Preheat your air fryer to 360f. Shape the mixture into cookie shapes and put them on a baking sheet that will sit 16 minutes or until cooked through in the air fryer bake.

Nutrition: calories

515 Fat9g

Carbs5g

Protein 4g

380) Pancakes nutellastuffed

Preparation time: 15 min

Cooking time: 20 min

Servings: 12 pancakes

Ingredients

Teaspoons of chocolate-hazelnut spread, such as nutella ®, at room temperature

1/4 cup vegetable oil, plus

1 1/4 cup grid all-purpose flour

1 1/4 cup buttermilk

1/4 cup of granulated sugar

One teaspoon baking soda

One teaspoon baking soda

One egg

A pinch of salt

Sugar for dusting

Maple syrup for serving

Line a parchment baking sheet and drop 12 different teaspoonful mounds of chocolate-hazelnut spread over it. Place the baking sheet on a counter to flatten the dollops and freeze for about 15 minutes until firm.

In the meantime, preheat a griddle over low heat and brush with oil lightly.

In a large bowl, whisk together the flour, buttermilk, oil, granulated sugar, baking powder, baking soda, egg and a pinch of salt until smooth.

Pour batter pools on the hot griddle and cook until bubbles just start forming on the pancakes surface and the bottoms are golden, 1 to 2 minutes. Place a frozen chocolate-hazelnut dish spread on 4 of the pancakes and flip the remaining four pancakes on top of those, so the wet batter envelopes the disks. Put the rest of the discs back into the freezer. Continue cooking the pancakes for about 1 minute, flipping halfway, until the edges are set. Repeat with the remaining batters and disks, oiling the grid lightly in between lots.

Stub the pancakes with the sugar of the confectioners and serve warmly with syrup.

Nutrition: calories

151 Fat9g

Carbs5g

Protein 4g

381) Air fryer banana bread

Preparation time: 15 min

Cooking time: 50 min

Servings: 4

Ingredients

Half cup all-purpose flour

1/4 cup wheat germ or whole-wheat flour

Half teaspoon kosher salt

1/4 teaspoon baking soda

Two ripe bananas

1/2 cup granulated sugar

1/4 cup vegetable oil

1/4 cup plain yogurt (not greek)

1/2 teaspoon pure vanilla extract

One large egg

1 to 2 tablespoons turbinate sugar, optional

Direction

Whisk together the flour, wheat germ, salt, and baking soda in a medium bowl. Mash the bananas in a separate medium bowl until very smooth. Fill the banana with the granulated sugar, oil, yogurt, vanilla, and egg and whisk until smooth. Sew the dry ingredients over the wet and fold with a spatula until just mixed together. Scrape the batter into an insert with 7 inches of round air fryer, metal cake pans or foil pan, and smooth the top. Sprinkle with the turbinate sugar on top of the batter if desired, for a crunchy, sweet topping.

Put the pan in a 5.3-quarter air fryer and cook at 310 degrees f until a toothpick inserted in the middle of the bread comes out clean, 30 to 35 minutes, turning the pan halfway through. Put the pan into a rack for 10 minutes to cool. Unmold the banana bread from the pan and let it cool down on the rack completely before slicing into wedges to serve.

Nutrition: calories

128 Fat9g

Carbs5g

Protein 4g

382) Air fryer shortbread recipe

Preparation time: 20 min

Cooking time: 60 min

Servings: 5

Ingredients:

250 g self-rising flour

175 g butter

75 g caster sugar

Additional ingredients:

30 g cocoa powder roses chocolates

2 tsp vanilla essence

Chocolate chips–imperial

Directions:

Put the flour, butter and caster sugar in a bowl. Apply the butter to the flour until thick breadcrumbs imitate it. Knead until you have a ball of shortbread dough

Shortbread is pure butter, sugar, and flour. The butter ties it together without the need for milk or eggs, because of the high level of butter.

It also saves washing up as you don't need a bowl for dry ingredients and a bowl for wet ingredients.

Next, the flour and sugar are added to the pot, and the fat is mixed into the meal. This makes incredibly thick breadcrumbs that will become a lovely soft shortbread with a bit of kneading, then roll it out and make whatever shapes you want, whether its fingers, circles, or using your made cutters for cookies.

It also gives you a regular shortbread cookie dough that you can use on a lot of different shortbread recipes.

Then you need your kitchen gadgets, of course: air fryer.

You can cook your shortbread cookies using either an air fryer grill pan or an air fryer baking sheet. It prevents them from sticking to the air fryer and ensures they cook flat place in a mixing bowl, your flour, sugar, and butter.

Rub the butter in the flour with your fingertips until you have moist breadcrumbs.

Knead into a ball, then roll with your cutters and form them.

Cook and serve warm.

Nutrition:

calories 175

Fat9g

Carbs5g

Protein 4g

383) Air fryer apple pie

There's just something about an apple pie baked fresh! The glorious cinnamon scent fills the air,

Preparation time: 10 mins

Cooking time: 30 mins

Servings: 3

Ingredients

1 pillsbury refrigerator crust baking spray

One large apple, chopped

Two teaspoons of lemon juice

One tablespoon of cinnamon

Two tablespoons of sugar

½ tablespoon of vanilla extract

One tablespoon of butter

One beaten egg

One tablespoon of raw sugar

Direction

Preheat the air fryer to the highest degree while the pie is being prepared.

Cut one crust about ⅛ inch larger than the pie, and a second one slightly smaller than the baking pan, using the smaller baking tin. To stretch the pie crust, you might need to roll the crust a tiny bit with a rollin plate. Set aside the smaller ones.

Sprinkle the baking tin with the spray and put the larger cut crust in the baking pan. Set aside.

Layer the chopped apple, lemon juice, cinnamon, sugar, and vanilla extract in a small bowl combine to blend.

Pour the apples with the pie crust into the baking saucepan.

Apple top with butter bits.

Place the second pie crust over the top and pinch the edge of the apples. Create several slits to the top of the dough.

Place beaten egg over the top of the crust and sprinkle on top of the egg mixture with raw sugar.

Place pie in a basket with air fryer.

Set the timer at 320 degrees for 30 minutes, when you preheat the air fryer; the air fryer works best for baked goods. Run air fryer empty while the food is being cooked at the highest temperature.

Serve two large parts or four small parts.

Nutrition:

calories 143

Fat9g

Carbs5g

Protein 4g

384) Air fryer chocolate cake

Preparation time: 10 minutes

Cooking time: 25 minutes

Servings: 4

Ingredients

Three eggs

1/2 cup sour cream

1 cup flour

2/3 cup sugar

One stick butter room temperature

1/3 cup cocoa powder

One teaspoon baking soda

1/2 teaspoon baking soda

Two teaspoons vanilla

Directions:

Preheat air fryer to 320 degrees mix low pour ingredients into oven attachment place in air fryer basket and slide into air fryer set timer to 25 minutes. Use a toothpick to see if the cake is made. Cook for another 5 minutes if it doesn't spring back when hit.

Nice cake on a wire rack coat with your favorite chocolate frosting

Nutrition:

calories 378

Fat9g

Carbs5g

Protein 4g

385) Tender sunflower cookies

Preparation time: 15 minutes

Cooking time: 10 minutes

Servings: 8

Ingredients:

5 oz. Sunflower seed butter

½ teaspoon salt

1 tablespoon stevia extract

6 tablespoon coconut flour

¼ teaspoon salt   ¼ teaspoon olive oil

Directions:

Combine the sunflower seed butter and coconut flour together.

Sprinkle the mixture with salt and stevia extract.

Add olive oil and mix it up.

When you get the homogeneous texture of the dough – it is done.

Separate the dough into 8 balls and flatten them gently.

Preheat the air fryer to 365 f.

Put the flattened balls in the air fryer rack.

Cook the cookies for 10 minutes.

When the cookies are cooked – let them cool well.

Enjoy! Nutrition:

calories 378 Fat9g

Carbs5g

Protein 4g

386) Keto chocolate spread

Preparation time: 10 minutes

Cooking time: 3 minutes

Servings: 6

Ingredients:

1 oz. Dark chocolate

3 oz. Hazelnuts, crushed

4 tablespoon butter

¼ cup almond milk

½ teaspoon vanilla extract

1 teaspoon stevia

Directions:

Preheat the air fryer to 360 f.

Put the dark chocolate, crushed hazelnuts, butter, almond milk, vanilla extract, and stevia in the air fryer basket.

Mix it up and cook for 2 minutes.

Then mix the mixture with the help of the hand mixer.

Cook the mixture for 1 minute.

Then stir the mixture again and pour it into the glass vessel.

Put the mixture in the fridge and let it cool until it is solid. Enjoy! Nutrition: calories 378 Fat9g

Carbs5g Protein 4g

387) Keto vanilla mousse

Preparation time: 15 minutes

Cooking time: 6 minutes

Servings: 4

Ingredients:

1 teaspoon vanilla extract

½ cup cream cheese

½ cup almond milk

¼ cup blackberries

2 teaspoon stevia extract

2 tablespoon butter ¼ teaspoon cinnamon

Directions:

Preheat the air fryer to 320 f.

Combine butter, vanilla extract, and almond milk and transfer the mixture in the air fryer.

Cook the mixture for 6 minutes or until the almond milk mixture will be homogenous.

Then stir it carefully and chill until the room temperature.

Smash the blackberries.

Whisk the cream cheese with the help of the hand whisker for 2 minutes.

Add the smashed blackberries and whisk for 1 minute more.

After this, add cinnamon and stevia extract.

Stir it gently.

Combine the almond-butter liquid and cream cheese mixture together.

Mix it up with the help of the hand mixer.

When the meal is homogenous – pour it into the glass vessel.

Place it in the fridge and cool.

Enjoy! Nutrition:
calories 378

Fat9g Carbs5g

Protein 4g

388) Avocado brownies

Preparation time: 15 minutes

Cooking time: 20 minutes

Servings: 6

Ingredients:

1avocado, pitted

2 teaspoon erythritol

¼ teaspoon vanilla extract

1 oz. Dark chocolate

3 tablespoon almond flour   ½ teaspoon stevia powder

1 egg

1 teaspoon coconut oil

¼ teaspoon baking powder

¼ teaspoon salt

Directions:

Peel the avocado and chop it roughly.

Put the chopped avocado in the blender.

Melt the dark chocolate and add it to the blender too.

After this, add vanilla extract and blend the mixture until it is smooth.

Then add almond flour, stevia powder, coconut oil, baking powder, salt, and erythritol.

Beat the egg in the mixture and blend it until smooth.

Preheat the air fryer to 355 f.

Pour the avocado brownie mixture in the air fryer tray and flatten it with the help of the spatula.

Cook the brownie dough for 20 minutes.

When the meal is cooked – cut it into 6 brownie bars and chill.

Enjoy! Nutrition:
calories 131 Fat9g

Carbs5g

Protein 4g

389) Chocolate chips cookies

Preparation time: 15 minutes

Cooking time: 15 minutes

Servings: 5

Ingredients:

1 cup almond flour

3 tablespoon macadamia nuts, crushed

1 egg

3 tablespoon butter, unsalted

2 tablespoon dark chocolate chips

¼ teaspoon salt

¼ teaspoon baking powder

½ teaspoon vanilla extract

1 teaspoon stevia extract

Directions:

Beat the egg in the mixing bowl and whisk it with the help of the hand whisker.

Add butter and almond flour.

After this, add salt, baking powder, vanilla extract, and stevia extract.

Sprinkle the mixture with the crushed macadamia nuts and dark chocolate chips.

Knead the smooth dough.

Then make 5 balls from the chocolate chips dough and flatten them little.

Preheat the air fryer to 360 f.

Put the cookies in the air fryer and cook them for 15 minutes.

After this, let the cooked cookies chill little.

Serve them!
Nutrition:
calories 157

Fat9g

Carbs5g

Protein 4g

390) Cheesecake mousse

Preparation time: 20 minutes

Cooking time: 4 minutes

Servings: 12

Ingredients:

¼ cup heavy cream
1 egg
½ cup cream cheese
1/3 cup erythritol
¼ teaspoon lime zest
2 scoop stevia

Directions:

Beat the egg in the mixer bowl and whisk it.

Add the heavy cream and keep whisking it until the mixture is fluffy.

Then add cream cheese, lime zest, stevia, and erythritol.

Whisk it well.

Preheat the air fryer to 310 f.

Pour the cheesecake mixture into the air fryer tray and cook it for 14 minutes.

Stir it every 4 minutes.

When the mousse is cooked – whisk it carefully with the help of the hand whisker.

Chill the meal and enjoy!

Nutrition:

calories 43

Fat9g

Carbs5g

Protein 4g

391) Sweet bacon cookies

Preparation time: 10 minutes

Cooking time: 7 minutes

Servings: 6

Ingredients:

4 slices bacon, cooked, chopped

5 tablespoon peanut butter

¼ teaspoon baking soda

3 tablespoon swerves

½ teaspoon vanilla extract   ¼ teaspoon ground ginger

Directions:

Take the big bowl and combine the baking soda, peanut butter, swerve, vanilla extract, and ground ginger together.

Add chopped bacon and mix the dough up with the help of the spatula.

When the dough is homogenous – make the log from it and cut it into 6 part.

Roll the balls from the dough and flatten them gently.

Preheat the air fryer to 350 f.

Place the cookies in the air fryer and cook for 7 minutes.

When the cookies are cooked – let them chill well.

Enjoy!

Nutrition: calories 109

Fat9g

Carbs5g

Protein 4g

392) Sunflower seeds pie

Preparation time: 20 minutes

Cooking time: 20 minutes

Servings: 6

Ingredients:

½ cup sunflower seeds

1 cup almond flour

¼ cup heavy cream

2 eggs

1 teaspoon butter

½ teaspoon vanilla extract ½ teaspoon ground ginger

3 scoop stevia

½ teaspoon baking powder
Directions:

Beat the eggs in the big bowl and whisk them.

Add heavy cream, butter, almond flour, vanilla extract, ground ginger, stevia, and baking powder.

Mix the dough mixture gently with the help of the hand mixer.

Then add the sunflower seeds and stir the dough with the help of the spatula.

Leave the pie dough for 10 minutes to rest.

Preheat the air fryer to 360 f.

Transfer the dough to the air fryer dish and place it in the preheated air fryer.

Cook the pie for 20 minutes.

Then let the pie chill well. After this, discard it from the air fryer dish and cut into servings. Enjoy!

Nutrition: calories 180 Fat9g

Carbs5g Protein 4g

393) Almond sponge cake

Preparation time: 15 minutes

Cooking time: 18 minutes

Servings: 6

Ingredients:

5 eggs

1 cup almond flour

¼ teaspoon salt

3 scoop stevia

Directions:

Separate the egg whites and egg yolks and place them in the separate bowls.

Then whisk the egg yolk for 3 minutes.

Add the stevia and whisk it for 1 minute more.

After this, whisk the egg whites until you get the strong peaks.

Combine the whisked egg yolks with the almond flour and salt.

Stir the mixture very slowly with the help of the spatula.

After this, start to add the egg white peaks in the egg yolk mixture gradually.

Stir it carefully until you get the fluffy yellow dough.

Preheat the air fryer to 280 f.

Pour the sponge cake dough in the air fryer tray and cook it for 18 minutes.

Check if the sponge cake is cooked with the help of the toothpick.

Chill the sponge cake carefully and discard it from the tray.

Serve the sponge cake with the small amount of the blueberries.

Enjoy!

Nutrition: calories 109

Fat9g

Carbs5g

Protein 4g

394) Blackberry pie

Preparation time: 15 minutes

Cooking time: 20 minutes

Servings: 8

Ingredients:

1 cup almond flour

2 tablespoon butter, unsalted

1 tablespoon baking powder

1 large egg

½ cup blackberries 1 scoop stevia extract

Directions:

Preheat the air fryer to 350 f.

Beat the egg in the bowl and whisk it.

Then add baking powder, stevia extract, and butter.

Mix it up.

Leave the 1 teaspoon almond flour.

Put all the remaining almond flour in the egg mixture.

Knead the smooth and non-sticky dough.

Cover the air fryer tray with the parchment.

Then put the dough in the air fryer dish and flatten it in the shape of the piecrust.

Place the blackberries over the piecrust.

Then sprinkle the pie with the 1 teaspoon of almond flour.

Cook the pie for 20 minutes.

When the surface of the pie is golden brown – it is cooked.

Chill it well and slice into the serving.

Enjoy!

Nutrition: calories 143

Fat9g

Carbs5g

Protein 4g

395) Coconut pie

Preparation time: 25 minutes

Cooking time: 10 minutes

Servings: 4

Ingredients:

1 cup almond flour
3 tablespoon butter
¼ teaspoon salt
1 scoop stevia
1 tablespoon ice water
3 eggs

½ cup heavy cream

1 teaspoon butter

2 tablespoon coconut flakes

1 teaspoon vanilla extract

Directions:

Preheat the air fryer to 360 f.

Combine the almond flour and 3 tablespoons of the butter in the bowl.

Add salt and stevia.

Blend it well.

When the mixture starts to be smooth – add ice water and blend it for 2 minutes more.

Cover the air fryer crust with the parchment and place the dough there.

Roll it with the help of the fingertips.

Place the piecrust in the air fryer and cook for 7 minutes.

Meanwhile, beat the eggs in the bowl and whisk them.

Add the 1 teaspoon of butter and heavy cream and whisk it well for 3 minutes.

Add coconut flakes and vanilla extract. Whisk it for 1 minute more.

When the piecrust is cooked – remove it from the air fryer and chill it.

Pour the whisked heavy cream mixture in the air fryer and cook it for 3 minutes at 365 f.

Then whisk it carefully.

Then pour the cooked heavy cream mixture over the piecrust.

Chill it until the filling of the pie is a little bit solid.

Serve it! Nutrition:
calories 109 Fat9g

Carbs5g

Protein 4g

396) Avocado muffins

Preparation time: 18 minutes

Cooking time: 12 minutes

Servings: 7

Ingredients:

1 oz. Dark chocolate, melted
1 cup almond flour
½ cup avocado, pitted
½ teaspoon baking soda
4 tablespoon butter

1 teaspoon apple cider vinegar
3 scoop stevia powder
1 egg

Directions:

Put the almond flour in the bowl.

Add baking soda and apple cider vinegar.

After this, add melted chocolate and stevia powder.

Crack the egg into the separate bowl and whisk it.

Add whisked egg in the almond flour mixture.

Add butter.

Then peel the avocado and mash it.

Add the mashed avocado in the almond flour mixture.

Use the hand mixer to make the almond flour mixture smooth and homogenous.

Preheat the air fryer to 355 f.

Pour the almond flour mixture in the muffin forms. Fill ½ part of every muffin mold.

Put the muffins in the air fryer and cook them for 9 minutes.

Then reduce the temperature to 340 f and cook the muffins for 3 minutes more.

Chill the cooked muffins and serve them!

Enjoy! Nutrition:
calories 136 Fat9g

Carbs5g

Protein 4g

397) Cream cheese muffins

Preparation time: 15 minutes

Cooking time: 10 minutes

Servings: 8

Ingredients:

1 egg

1 cup cream cheese

1 cup almond flour

¼ teaspoon salt

1 teaspoon baking soda

1 teaspoon apple cider vinegar

2 teaspoon swerves 2 tablespoon coconut flakes

Directions:

Beat the egg in the bowl and add cream cheese.

Whisk the mixture well.

Sprinkle the cream cheese mixture with the almond flour, salt, baking soda, and apple cider vinegar.

Add swerve and coconut flakes.

Use the hand mixer to make the sour cream-like dough.

Preheat the air fryer to 360 f.

Fill the ½ part of every muffin mold with the muffin dough and put the muffins in the air fryer.

Cook the muffins for 10 minutes.

When the muffins are cooked – let them chill well.

Then serve.

Taste it!

Nutrition: calories 124

Fat9g

Carbs5g

Protein 4g

398) Cream pie with lemon

Preparation time: 20 minutes

Cooking time: 21 minutes

Servings: 8

Ingredients:

1 lemon

1cup heavy cream

2 eggs

3 tablespoon butter

1 teaspoon baking soda

3 tablespoon coconut flour

1 ½ cup almond flour

2 teaspoon swerves

1 scoop stevia

¼ teaspoon salt

Directions:

Wash the lemon and slice it into the thin rings.

Beat the eggs in the blender.

Add heavy cream, butter, and baking soda.

Blend it well on the maximum speed for 2 minutes.

After this, add coconut flour, almond flour, swerve, and salt.

Blend the mixture for 3 minutes more.

The blended dough should be smooth but non-sticky.

Preheat the air fryer to 300 f.

Place the parchment in the air fryer dish.

Roll the dough with the help of the rolling pin and transfer it to the air fryer dish.

Then place the sliced lemon over the piecrust.

Sprinkle the pie with the stevia.

Cook the pie for 21 minutes.

When the pie is cooked – chill it until the room temperature.

Cut it into the servings.

Taste it! Nutrition:
calories 109 Fat9g

Carbs5g

Protein 4g

399) Raspberry cobbler

Preparation time: 15 minutes

Cooking time: 10 minutes

Servings: 6

Ingredients:

1 cup raspberries
1 cup almond flour
1 tablespoon butter, melted
1 egg
½ teaspoon vanilla extract
2 teaspoon stevia powder

Directions:

Preheat the air fryer to 360 f.

Slice and put the raspberries in the air fryer dish.

Sprinkle the berries with 1 teaspoon of stevia powder.

Combine the almond flour, butter, and vanilla extract in the bowl.

Beat the egg in the almond flour and stir it carefully until homogenous.

Then place the homogenous almond mixture over the sliced raspberries.

Sprinkle the dough with the 1 teaspoon of the stevia powder.

Put the cobbler in the air fryer dish. Cover the cobbler with the foil and make the x cut in the center of the foil.

Then cook it for 10 minutes.

If it is raw – cook it for 2-3 minutes more till it gets the doneness level.

Cut the cobbler and serve.

Enjoy! Nutrition:
calories 109 Fat9g

Carbs5g

Protein 4g

400) Vanilla-cinnamon cookies

Preparation time: 15 minutes

Cooking time: 10 minutes

Servings: 14

Ingredients:

1 egg
1 tablespoon ground cinnamon
1 teaspoon vanilla extract

2 teaspoon-swerve

1 scoop stevia powder

1 teaspoon baking soda

1 teaspoon apple cider vinegar

2 tablespoon coconut flour

1 cup almond flour

2 tablespoon heavy cream

¼ teaspoon salt 3
tablespoon butter

Directions:

Crack the egg in the blender and blend it until smooth.

Then add ground cinnamon, vanilla extract, swerve, stevia powder, baking   soda, and apple   cider vinegar.

Blend the mixture for 30 seconds.

Then add coconut flour, almond flour, heavy cream, salt, and butter. Blend the mixture for 2 minutes.

You will get the soft and elastic dough.

Roll the dough and make the cookies from it with the help of the cutter.

Preheat the air fryer to 355 f.

Cover the air fryer dish with the parchment and put the cookies there.

Cook the cookies for 10 minutes.

Then let the cookies cool well.

Enjoy! Nutrition:
calories 90 Fat9g

Carbs5g

Protein 4g

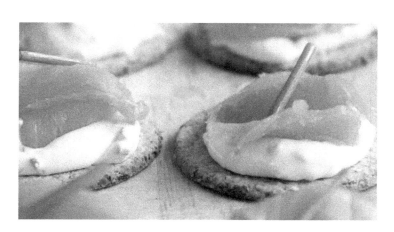

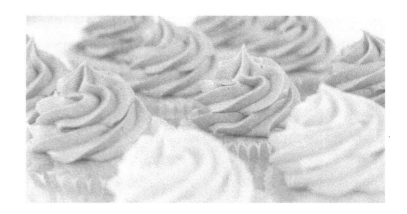

Conclusion

Living the keto lifestyle can be tough, but only if you allow it to be.

Counting your carbohydrates

Measuring your carb intake is extremely important and should never be neglected. Being lackadaisical about doing this in time will become a part of your routine, and that would eventually defeat the aim of the dieting. So, in order to prevent this, you need to constantly read the labels on foods you're having and ensure that the carbohydrates proportions are suitable for your daily allowance. Whenever you are out in a grocery store, ensure you read the labels on everything you purchase. Undeniably, it may be burdensome, but it will be worth it in the end. When deciding the carb count in foods, calculate the net carbs (net carbs = total carbs – fiber).

Your goal should be to consume about 20 net carbs per day. It is perfectly alright if there are substitutes, but the rule is to consume an intake of 20 to 35 net carbs a day. But if you are exercising, it is advisable that you eat your daily net carbs before you begin exercising as your body will burn glucose during the exercise and revert to using ketones subsequently. Having a small carb intake before exercising is an excellent idea to acquiring some quick energy into your body so that you can take your workout all the way.

Make sure that during your first months, you maintain a record of what you are consuming daily. Sometimes it can be a mere blunder or a snack that drives you over the carb threshold.

Clean out your kitchen

Many people fall to the temptation of food quite easily. Do your best not to be one of them. Do away with any food that is high in carbohydrates in your kitchen or refrigerator; this is especially the case in candies, chocolates, caffeine, sodas, juices, bread, gluten, pasta, rice, potatoes, etc. If you don't want to throw away all these foods, simply give it to a friend, family member, neighbor, or donate.

After that, head to the grocery store, execute your new label reading tactics and renew your fridge and pantry with low-carb options to feed on. Believe me; you will feel better about this once your food addictions are conquered

Keto diets and restaurants

When you begin a keto-friendly lifestyle, be mindful of what kind of diners and restaurants you are going to. You may want to go over an online menu in advance, so you know exactly what you'll get and have the carb count. In due course, you can order from menus in restaurants you have never gone in before as you can calculate the net carbs in every recipe. Below are some ketogenic-friendly orders you can find in almost all restaurants:

For breakfast: eggs, bacon, and sausage.

For lunch: chicken salad (without salad dressings)

For dinner: meat!

Eating low carb actively

Fast foods, snacks, and cravings will always be present in our lives. Be sure to have your refrigerator and pantry stored with snacks to eat if you're in a rush or starving. If you have works to do, ensure you pack your lunch in advance along with a snack.

Now, strict adherence to these steps will assure you of a higher chance of attaining a successful ketogenic diet journey!

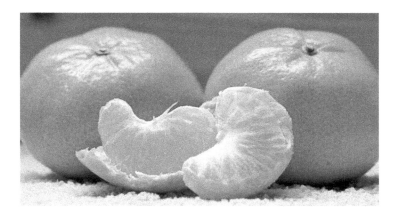

CPSIA information can be obtained
at www.ICGtesting.com
Printed in the USA
LVHW102159110121
676251LV00041B/641